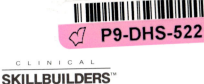

C L I N I C A L
SKILLBUILDERS™

Diagnostic Test Implications

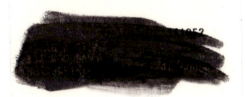

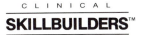

CLINICAL
SKILLBUILDERS™

Diagnostic Test Implications

Springhouse Corporation
Springhouse, Pennsylvania

STAFF

Executive Director, Editorial
Stanley Loeb

Editorial Director
Matthew Cahill

Clinical Director
Barbara F. McVan, RN

Art Director
John Hubbard

Senior Editor
William J. Kelly

Clinical Project Editor
Judith A. Schilling McCann, RN, BSN

Editors
Barbara Delp, Margaret Eckman, Kevin Law, Elizabeth Mauro

Clinical Editors
Lynore DeSilets, RN, EdD; Maryann Foley, RN, BSN; Mary Gyetvan, RN, BSEd

Copy Editors
Jane V. Cray (supervisor), Nancy Papsin, Doris Weinstock

Designers
Stephanie Peters (associate art director), Matie Patterson (senior designer), Linda Franklin

Illustrators
Jean Gardner, Robert Jackson, Robert Neumann, Judy Newhouse, Robert Phillips

Art Production
Robert Perry (manager), Anna Brindisi, Donald Knauss, Thomas Robbins, Robert Wieder

Typography
David Kosten (director), Diane Paluba (manager), Elizabeth Bergman, Joyce Rossi Biletz, Phyllis Marron, Robin Rantz, Valerie Rosenberger

Manufacturing
Deborah Meiris (manager), T.A. Landis, Jennifer Suter

Production Coordination
Colleen M. Hayman

Editorial Assistants
Maree DeRosa, Beverly Lane, Mary Madden

Library of Congress Cataloging-in-Publication Data

Diagnostic test implications.
      p.   cm. – (Clinical Skillbuilders)
    Includes bibliographical references and index.
    1. Diagnosis, Laboratory.   2. Function tests (Medicine).   3. Nursing.   I. Springhouse Corporation. II. Series.
      [DNLM: 1. Diagnosis – nurses' instruction. 2. Nursing Care.   WY 100 D5348]
    RB37.D493   1991
    616.07'5 – dc20
    DNLM/DLC   91-4738
    for Library of Congress   CIP
    ISBN 0-87434-380-1

CONTENTS

ADVISORY BOARD AND CONTRIBUTORS

At the time of publication, the advisors held the following positions.

Sandra G. Crandall, RN,C, MSN, CRNP
Director
Center for Nursing Excellence
Newtown, Pa.

Ellen Eggland, RN, MN
Vice President
Healthcare Personnel, Inc.
Naples, Fla.

Terry Matthew Foster, RN, BSN, CCRN, CEN
Clinical Director, Nursing Administration
Mercy Hospital – Anderson
Cincinnati
Staff Nurse, Emergency Department
St. Elizabeth Medical Center
Covington, Ky.

Sandra K. Goodnough-Hanneman, RN, PhD
Critical Care Nursing Consultant
Houston

Doris A. Millam, RN, MS, CRNI
I.V. Therapy Clinician
Holy Family Hospital
Des Plaines, Ill.

Deborah Panozzo Nelson, RN, MS, CCRN
Cardiovascular Clinical Specialist
Visiting Assistant Professor
EMS Nursing Education
Purdue University, Calumet Campus
Hammond, Ind.

Sally S. Russell, RN, MN, CS
Instructor
Clinical Specialist
St. Elizabeth Hospital Medical Center
Lafayette, Ind.

Marilyn Sawyer Sommers, RN, PhD, CCRN
Nurse Consultant
Instructor
College of Nursing and Health
University of Cincinnati

At the time of publication, the contributors held the following positions.

Emmie J. Amerine, RN, BS
Clinical Coordinator
Offices of James R. Bollinger, MD
Paoli, Pa.

Marjorie Davis Beck, RN
Nurse Manager, Gastrointestinal Procedures Unit
Abington (Pa.) Memorial Hospital

Barbara Anne Boston, RN
Head Nurse, Cardiac Catheterization Unit
Hahnemann University Hospital
Philadelphia

Heather Boyd-Monk, SRN, BSN, CRNO
Assistant Director of Nursing for Education Programs
Wills Eye Hospital
Philadelphia

Marlene Ciranowicz, RN, MSN, CDE
Independent Nurse Consultant
Dresher, Pa.

Paulette Dorney, RN, MSN, CCRN
Clinical Instructor
Lehigh County Community College
Schnecksville, Pa.
Staff Nurse, Critical Care
Easton (Pa.) Hospital

Bonita Ann Giordano, RN, BSN
Staff Nurse, OB/GYN Center
Abington (Pa.) Memorial Hospital

Karen A. Graf, RN, BSN, CURN
Urology Nurse Coordinator
Rusk Institute of Rehabilitation Medicine
New York University Medical Center

Mary Gyetvan, RN, BSEd
Independent Nurse Consultant
Levittown, Pa.

Mary Faut Rodts, RN, MS, ONC
Assistant Professor
Rush University College of Nursing
Chicago

Donald A. St. Onge, RN, MSN
Pulmonary Clinical Specialist
Allegheny General Hospital
Pittsburgh, Pa.

Julie N. Tackenburg, RN, MA, CNRN
Clinical Nurse Specialist
University Medical Center
Tucson, Ariz.

FOREWORD

In today's world of high-tech health care, diagnostic tests play an increasingly important role. And keeping pace with what you need to know about sophisticated diagnostic tests (and even some fairly simple ones) poses quite a challenge.

After all, you must understand why and how diagnostic tests are performed so you can prepare your patients beforehand and care for them afterward. In some cases, you also need to know how to collect a specimen, perform a bedside test, or assist the doctor with the procedure. And just as important, you must know how to alter your nursing care if test results turn out to be abnormal.

Diagnostic Test Implications, the latest volume in the Clinical Skillbuilders series, will help you learn all that and more. The book focuses on what nurses need to know about approximately 125 of the most common diagnostic tests.

Chapter 1 covers a wide range of blood, urine, and fecal studies—from routine urinalysis to the HIV antibody serum enzyme immunoassay. In the introduction to this chapter, you'll find detailed instructions on how to collect the various specimens for the tests. Chapter 2 covers common culture studies, including nasopharyngeal and throat cultures. Chapter 3 discusses biopsies, and Chapter 4, radiographic studies, such as computed tomography, mammography, and plain X-rays.

In Chapter 5, you'll read about nuclear scans, such as cardiac blood pool imaging and the T_3 thyroid suppression test. Chapter 6 covers ultrasound studies, including Doppler ultrasonography and echocar-

diography, and Chapter 7 addresses common endoscopic procedures. In Chapter 8, the discussion turns to special studies, such as electrocardiography, magnetic resonance imaging, and pulmonary function tests.

To save you time when looking up key information, each test follows the same format. Each begins with a brief introduction, covering such topics as how the test works and why it's used. Next comes a quick listing of the test's specific diagnostic purposes. Then you'll find a thorough explanation of your role before, during, and after the procedure.

The next two sections spell out the normal results for the test and the medical implications of abnormal results, respectively. But it's the final section that makes *Diagnostic Test Implications* especially useful. In this section, you'll read about the *nursing* implications of abnormal results. Here the authors tell you how to provide nursing care based on the results of your patient's diagnostic test.

Throughout the book, special graphic devices, or logos, signal helpful sidebars. The *Checklist* logo, for instance, refers you to listings of key information. In Chapter 1, this logo accompanies a list of safeguards for performing venipunctures. The *Complications* logo signals information on identifying and managing complications associated with a procedure. And whenever you see a *Procedures* logo, you'll discover an explanation of how to perform or assist with a particular procedure.

Near the back of the book you'll find a multiple-choice self-test designed to help you evaluate how much you've learned and further build your skills. An answer key follows the last question. After this self-test comes an important appendix listing drugs that interfere with the results of common laboratory tests.

Packed with practical clinical information, this book is a must for today's nurse. Whether you are just starting your career or have been practicing for years, it will update, clarify, and expand your role in diagnostic tests. I recommend that you review *Diagnostic Test Implications*, then take it to work and keep it close at hand.

Joyce Wolf Roth, RN, MSN, CCRN
Coordinator, Nursing Education
New York Hospital

1

BLOOD, URINE, AND FECAL STUDIES

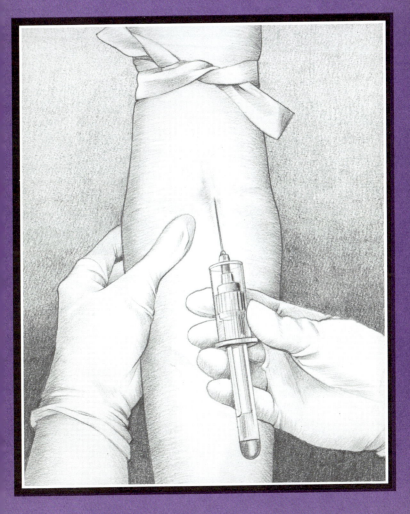

Despite the many technological advances in diagnostic equipment and techniques, blood, urine, and fecal studies remain among the most common and most important diagnostic tests. And because you play a direct role in carrying them out, your knowledge and skill significantly influence the accuracy of the results.

To carry out your role, you need a basic understanding of these tests — their purposes, your part in the procedures, and your interventions after you receive the test results. In this chapter, you'll find such essential information for the most important blood, urine, and fecal studies you'll encounter.

The chapter begins by describing the procedures you'll use to collect blood, urine, and fecal samples. Then come explanations of the individual tests. For each test, you'll find a brief description; the test's purpose; procedure-related nursing care; reference values and abnormal results; and the implications of abnormal results on your nursing care.

When collecting a sample for any of these tests, wear gloves to protect yourself from infection should you come in contact with any body fluids.

Blood studies

Among the most common diagnostic procedures, blood studies serve several purposes. A doctor may order a blood study as part of a routine physical examination or an admission procedure. He also may order a blood study as a screening tool, or he may use it to confirm a suspected diagnosis.

Blood studies can be divided into three basic types — hematologic, blood chemistry, and immunologic tests. Hematologic tests, such as hemoglobin studies, analyze blood components and the process of hemostasis. Blood chemistry tests analyze numerous chemical substances found in the body, providing clues to how well major body systems are functioning. Such tests include electrolyte, enzyme, lipid, hormone, glucose, protein, and bile pigment studies. Immunologic tests, such as screening for the human immunodeficiency virus antibody, evaluate immune responses.

Collection techniques. The type of blood sample, the collection site, and the technique will depend on the test itself as well as on the patient's age and condition.

Venous sample. Most blood tests require a venous sample, often collected by laboratory personnel. If you're collecting the sample, make sure you perform the venipuncture carefully to reduce the risk of vein damage and hematoma formation and to diminish the patient's discomfort. (See *Safeguards for venipuncture.*)

Before the procedure, label the collection tubes clearly with the patient's name and room number, the doctor's name, and the date and time of collection. Then select a venipuncture site. The most common site is the antecubital fossa. Other sites include the wrist and the dorsum of the hand or foot. (See *Common arterial and venous puncture sites,* page 4.)

Next, position the patient on his back with his arms at his sides and his head slightly elevated. You can have an ambulatory patient sit on a chair.

If you're using a syringe, attach the needle to the barrel. If you're using an evacuated tube, attach the needle to the holder. Then tie a soft rubber tourniquet above the venipuncture site to make the patient's veins more prominent. (You may not need to do this if the patient already has prominent veins.) Instruct the patient to make a fist several times to further enlarge the veins. Then use inspection and palpation to select a vein.

Working in a circular motion from the center outward, clean the puncture site with alcohol or povidone-iodine solution. Allow the skin to dry. Then put on clean gloves, wipe the fingertips with an antiseptic, and palpate the vein again. To keep the vein from moving, draw the skin tautly over the vein and press just below the puncture site with your thumb.

Now, hold the syringe or evacuated tube so that the bevel of the needle is up and the shaft is parallel to the path of the vein at a 15-degree angle to the arm. Gently insert the needle into the vein.

If you're using a syringe, watch for dark red blood in the hub. Then gently pull back on the plunger to create suction, drawing in the desired amount of blood. If you're using an evacuated tube, look for a drop of blood just inside the needle holder. Once you see it, push the evacuated tube into the holder so that the end of the needle punctures the rubber stopper on the top of the evacuated tube. (See *Guide to color-top collection tubes,* page 5.) Blood will automatically flow into the tube. If you need more than one sample, repeat the procedure with another evacuated tube.

Release the tourniquet as soon as you've established an adequate blood flow. Once you've drawn up all the blood you need, ask the patient to open his fist. Cover the puncture site with a gauze pad, and slowly and gently withdraw the needle. To prevent a hematoma, apply

Safeguards for venipuncture

Follow these guidelines to protect your patient during venipuncture.
☐ Take precautions to ensure that the patient won't fall should syncope develop. Have him lie down or, if you have him sit, be ready to support him.
☐ If possible, don't draw blood from an arm or leg being used for an I.V. infusion of blood, dextrose, or electrolytes. These solutions will dilute the blood sample. If you must use a limb that's receiving an infusion, choose a location distal to the I.V. site.
☐ To identify veins more easily in a patient with tortuous or sclerosed veins or with veins damaged by repeated venipunctures, antibiotic therapy, or chemotherapy, apply warm, wet compresses 15 minutes before the procedure.
☐ When using a syringe, make sure the plunger is fully depressed before you insert the needle. This helps ensure that you don't inject air into a vein.
☐ If you aren't successful after two attempts, ask another nurse to perform the venipuncture.
☐ If you can't find a vein quickly, release the tourniquet temporarily to avoid tissue necrosis and circulation problems.
☐ Make sure you insert the needle at the correct angle to reduce the risk of puncturing the opposite wall of the vein and causing a hematoma.
☐ Always release the tourniquet before withdrawing the needle to prevent a hematoma. When drawing multiple samples, release the tourniquet within 1 minute of beginning to draw blood to prevent a hemoconcentrated sample.

light pressure to the puncture site until bleeding stops—usually in 2 to 3 minutes. The patient can do this if he's alert and cooperative. Then

Common arterial and venous puncture sites

This illustration shows the most common sites for collecting arterial and venous blood samples. Arterial sites are shown on the right side of the body; venous sites, on the left.

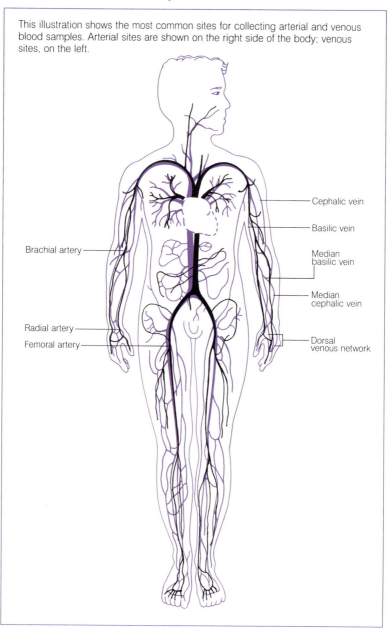

cover the site with a small adhesive bandage.

If you used a syringe, remove the needle and carefully empty the sample into the appropriate test tube. Don't eject the blood through the needle or force it out of the syringe. Doing so could cause foaming and hemolysis.

If the tube contains an additive (such as an anticoagulant), gently invert it several times to mix the sample thoroughly. Don't shake the tube, or you may cause hemolysis. Examine the sample for clots or clumps. If you don't see any, send the sample to the laboratory immediately.

Following hospital policy, dispose of the needle. Remove and discard your gloves and wash your hands.

Before leaving the patient, check his condition. If a hematoma has developed at the puncture site, apply warm soaks. If the patient has lingering discomfort or undue bleeding, tell him to lie down. Observe him for anxiety and signs of shock, such as hypotension and tachycardia.

Arterial sample. Rarely required for routine studies, arterial blood samples may be collected by a doctor or a specially trained nurse. These samples may be drawn directly from the radial, brachial, or femoral artery, or they may be drawn from an arterial line.

Before collecting an arterial sample, obtain an arterial blood pressure kit and fill the enclosed specimen bag with ice. If you're using an unheparinized syringe, attach a 20G needle to the syringe, break open the ampule of heparin, and draw 1 ml into the syringe. Then pull the plunger back past the 7-ml mark while rotating the barrel. Next, hold the syringe upright and

Guide to color-top collection tubes

Use this guide to select the correct tube for collecting a venous blood sample.
☐ *Red-top* tubes contain no additives. Use them for serum samples.
☐ *Lavender-top* tubes contain EDTA. Use them for whole blood samples.
☐ *Green-top* tubes contain heparin. Use them for certain plasma samples.
☐ *Blue-top* tubes contain sodium citrate and citric acid. Use them to collect plasma samples for coagulation studies.
☐ *Black-top* tubes contain sodium oxalate. Like blue-top tubes, use them to collect plasma samples for coagulation studies.
☐ *Gray-top* tubes contain a glycolysis inhibitor. Use them to collect serum or plasma samples for glucose determinations.

slowly force the heparin toward the hub as you continue rotating the barrel. Leave just enough heparin to fill the syringe tip. About 0.1 ml should suffice.

To collect a sample directly from an artery: First, heparinize the needle. To do so, replace the 20G needle with a 23G one. Holding the syringe upright but slightly tilted, push the plunger all the way up to eject the remaining heparin. Cap the needle and set the syringe aside.

The preferred puncture site is usually the radial artery. But before performing a radial artery puncture, you must use Allen's test to check the patency of the ulnar artery (see *Performing Allen's test,* pages 6 and 7). You won't perform a radial puncture unless the ulnar artery can provide an adequate blood supply to the hand. If you can't use either ra-

Performing Allen's test

Before drawing a sample from the radial artery, make sure the ulnar artery alone can supply the hand with blood in case a problem develops.

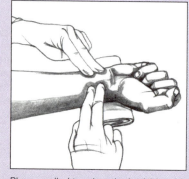

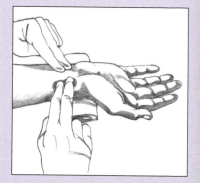

Place a rolled towel on the bedside table and have the patient rest his wrist on it. Then ask him to make a fist. Exert pressure on the radial and ulnar arteries with your middle and index fingers.

Ask the patient to unclench his fist. You'll notice that his palm is blanched because you've impaired the normal blood flow with your fingers.

dial artery, consider using the brachial artery. Because of the risk of severe bleeding, use the femoral artery only when circulation through the radial and brachial arteries is inadequate.

Once you've determined the appropriate site, put on clean gloves. Working in a circular motion from the center outward, clean the puncture site with an antiseptic wipe. Let the skin dry. Then wipe your gloved index finger with an antiseptic wipe and palpate the artery. Hold the syringe over the puncture site with the other hand.

With the needle bevel up, puncture the skin at a 45-degree angle for the radial artery and at a 60-degree angle for the brachial artery. If you need to use the femoral artery,

hold the needle at a 90-degree angle. Advance the needle, but don't pull the plunger back. The blood will pulsate into the syringe on its own. Allow 5 to 10 ml to enter the syringe.

If the syringe doesn't fill immediately, you may have pushed the needle through the artery. Pull the needle back slightly, remembering not to pull the plunger back. If the syringe still doesn't fill, withdraw the needle and start over with a fresh heparinized needle. Never make more than two attempts to draw blood from the same site.

After drawing the sample, remove the needle and apply firm pressure to the puncture site with a gauze pad for at least 5 minutes — 10 minutes for the larger femoral artery —

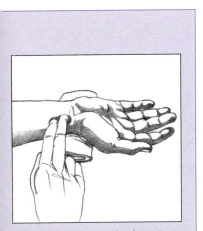

Release the pressure on the ulnar artery. If it can provide an adequate blood supply, the palm will turn pink in about 5 seconds. But if blood return is slow and the fingers begin to contract, blood supply from the ulnar artery isn't adequate.

to prevent a hematoma, a significant risk after arterial puncture. If the patient is receiving an anticoagulant or has a bleeding disorder, apply pressure for at least 15 minutes. Don't ask the patient to apply pressure to the site. He may not apply the necessary continuous, firm pressure.

To collect a sample from an arterial line: Put on clean gloves. Then eject the remaining heparin from the syringe and set it aside. Locate the stopcock attached to the arterial line and remove the cap from the closed outlet. Attach a 3- to 5-ml unheparinized syringe to the outlet, and turn the stopcock to close off the infusion and open the outlet to the syringe. After allowing the syringe to fill with blood, turn the

stopcock to close all outlets and remove the blood-filled syringe. This sample is contaminated with infusate, so you won't be able to use it for arterial blood gas studies.

Next, attach the heparinized syringe to the outlet. Turn the stopcock to open the outlet to the syringe and allow arterial blood to fill the syringe. Once you've collected the sample, turn the stopcock to close all outlets. Remove the syringe and cap the port. Then restart the infusion and adjust the flow rate as necessary. Attach a needle to the syringe.

Once you've collected the sample, either directly from the artery or from the arterial line, rotate the syringe to mix the heparin with the sample. If air bubbles appear, try to remove them by holding the syringe upright and tapping it lightly with your finger. If the bubbles don't disappear, remove them by holding the syringe upright, piercing a 2″ x 2″ gauze pad or alcohol swab with the needle, and slowly forcing some of the blood out of the syringe to eliminate the bubbles. The gauze pad will catch the blood. (If you can't remove the air bubbles because you're still applying pressure to the arterial puncture site, ask another nurse to do this.) After removing any air bubbles, slide the needle into a rubber stopper to seal it from the air, and put the syringe into the bag of ice.

If you've been applying pressure on the puncture site, release the pressure, check for bleeding, and tape a bandage firmly over the site.

Remove and discard your gloves and wash your hands. Note the patient's temperature, hemoglobin level, and the type and amount of oxygen he's receiving on the laboratory slip. Send the sample to the laboratory.

After an arterial puncture, monitor the patient for signs and symptoms of circulatory impairment distal to the puncture site. These include swelling, discoloration, pain, numbness, and tingling.

Capillary sample. To collect this sample, you'll need to puncture the patient's fingertip or earlobe. With a neonate, you'll use the great toe or heel.

Select the puncture site, avoiding cold, cyanotic, or swollen areas. Then apply warm, moist compresses to the area for about 10 minutes. This dilates the capillaries, helping ensure an adequate sample. Wipe the site with a gauze pad soaked in alcohol. Then dry the site thoroughly with another alcohol pad.

Put on clean gloves, select a lancet smaller than 2 mm, and puncture the skin. For a fingertip sample, make the puncture perpendicular to the lines of the patient's fingerprints.

When the first drop of blood appears, wipe it away to reduce the chance of diluting the sample with tissue fluid. For the same reason, you should avoid squeezing the puncture site. Then collect the sample.

Briefly apply pressure to the puncture site to prevent painful extravasation of blood. Ask an adult patient to hold a sterile gauze pad over the puncture site until the bleeding has stopped. Then apply a small adhesive bandage. Remove and discard your gloves and wash your hands.

Urine studies

Besides providing information about renal and urinary function, urine studies serve as sensitive indicators of overall health. In many cases, they're used to begin a diagnostic workup. A doctor may also order urine studies to monitor the levels of specific substances, including hormones, electrolytes, and glucose.

Collection techniques. The type of specimen required — clean-catch, second-voided, or timed — depends on the patient's condition and age and the test's purpose. You may need to collect the sample from a catheter if the patient can't void voluntarily or has an indwelling catheter in place. With an infant, you'll use the same basic collection procedure for all urine specimens. (See *Collecting a urine specimen from an infant.*)

Whether you're collecting a clean-catch, second-voided, or timed specimen, carefully explain the procedure to the patient. Tell him not to include toilet tissue or stool in any urine specimen because doing so can alter the test results.

After collecting the specimen, label the container with the patient's name and room number, the type of specimen, the collection time and, if possible, the suspected diagnosis. Send the specimen to the laboratory immediately.

Clean-catch specimen collection. Originally used primarily to test for bacteriuria and pyuria, this has become the method of choice for obtaining a random specimen because it's aseptic. To collect the specimen, ask the patient to thoroughly clean his perineal area. Tell him to then start voiding, into either a bedpan or toilet, and to collect a specimen in midstream.

Second-voided specimen collection. This method provides a specimen that isn't concentrated and thus more accurately reflects urine components. To collect this specimen,

Collecting a urine specimen from an infant

To collect a urine specimen from an infant, first thoroughly clean and dry the perineal area. Then apply the plastic urine collection bag. For a boy, apply the bag over the penis and scrotum, pressing the bag's flaps against the perineum to ensure a tight fit, as shown. For a girl, hold the legs apart as shown and apply the device to the perineum, starting at the point between the anus and the vagina and working toward the front. Place a diaper over the collection bag to keep the infant from tampering with it.

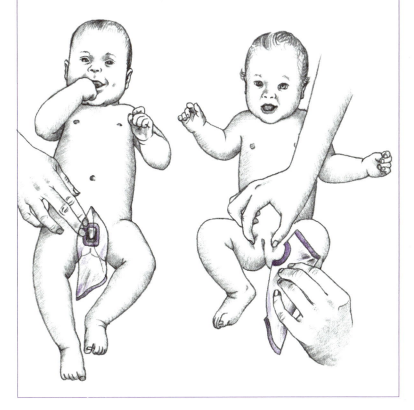

tell the patient to void and discard the urine, then void again 30 minutes later into a clean, dry specimen container, bedpan, or urinal.

Timed specimen collection. This method is used to determine the levels of such substances as hormones, proteins, creatinine, and electrolytes over a specified period—usually 2, 12, or 24 hours. To collect the specimen, have the patient void and discard the urine, then begin the timed collection with the next voiding. Emphasize to him that he must collect all urine during the test period. Just before the end of this period, have him void and add that specimen to the container. During the test period, you may need to add a preservative to the urine container and refrigerate it or keep it on ice.

Collection with a straight catheter. Although this method increases the risk of bacterial infection in the lower genitourinary tract, you may need to use it to collect a specimen from a patient who can't void voluntarily.

First, put on sterile gloves and, using sterile technique, catheterize the patient. Let a few milliliters of urine drain into a basin. Then, depending on test requirements, collect 10 to 60 ml of urine in a sterile plastic container.

Once you've collected enough urine, remove the catheter. Clean the area and let it dry. Then remove and discard your gloves and wash your hands.

Collection from an indwelling urinary catheter. When a patient has an indwelling catheter, clamp the collection tube about 30 minutes before collecting the specimen. Just before collecting the specimen, put on clean gloves.

If the collection tube has a sampling port, wipe it with an alcohol swab, insert a 22G needle at a 90-degree angle, and aspirate the urine into the syringe. If the tube doesn't have a port but the catheter is made of self-sealing rubber, you can collect the specimen from the catheter. To do so, wipe the catheter with an alcohol swab just above the connection of the collection tube to the catheter. Then insert a needle into the catheter at a 45-degree angle

and withdraw the urine specimen. Don't use this technique on silicone or plastic catheters; they'll leak after you withdraw the needle. And never insert the needle into the shaft of the catheter or you may puncture the lumen leading to the balloon.

After collecting the specimen, unclamp the tube and transfer the specimen to a sterile container. Remove and dispose of your gloves, and wash your hands.

Note: Don't use this procedure on patients who have just undergone genitourinary surgery.

Fecal studies

You may receive an order to collect a stool specimen for a few different tests. One of the most common is the test for fecal occult blood.

Collection technique. Because stool specimens can't be obtained on demand, you'll need to instruct the patient carefully beforehand. Warn him not to contaminate the specimen with urine or toilet tissue. And tell him to let you know when he has the urge to defecate.

When he's ready, have him defecate into a clean, dry bedpan. Then put on clean gloves and use a tongue blade to transfer a specimen from the bedpan to a container. Include any blood, mucus, or pus the patient has passed with the stool. Cap the container.

Remove your gloves and wash your hands thoroughly to prevent cross-contamination. Wrap the tongue blade in a paper towel and discard it.

Label the specimen container with the patient's name and room number and the date and time of collection. Then send it to the laboratory. If the specimen can't be transported immediately, refrigerate it.

Make sure the patient is comfortable after the procedure and that he has a chance to thoroughly clean his hands and perianal area. With some patients, you may need to perform perineal care.

Activated partial thromboplastin time

The activated partial thromboplastin time (APTT) test evaluates all the clotting factors of the intrinsic pathway, except Factor VII and Factor XIII. It measures the time needed to form a fibrin clot after calcium and phospholipid emulsion are added to a plasma sample, relying on an activator, such as kaolin, to shorten clotting time.

Because most congenital coagulation deficiencies occur in the intrinsic pathway, the APTT test serves as a preoperative screening for bleeding tendencies. It's also the test of choice for monitoring heparin therapy.

Purpose
• To screen for deficiencies of the clotting factors in the intrinsic pathway (except Factor VII and Factor XIII)
• To monitor heparin therapy.

Procedure-related nursing care
Explain the test's purpose to the patient and tell him the test requires a blood sample. Inform a patient who's receiving heparin therapy that the test may be repeated at regular intervals to assess his response to treatment.

Perform a venipuncture, collecting a blood sample in a 7-ml blue-top tube.

Reference values
A fibrin clot should form 25 to 36 seconds after a reagent is added.

Abnormal results
A prolonged APTT may indicate a deficiency of certain plasma clotting factors or the presence of heparin, fibrin split products, fibrinolysin, or circulating anticoagulants that act as antibodies to specific clotting factors.

Nursing implications of abnormal results
Monitor a patient with a prolonged APTT for bruising, nosebleeds, hematuria, and tarry stools. Regularly check his hemoglobin level, hematocrit, and platelet count. A decreased hemoglobin level or hematocrit could indicate bleeding; a decreased platelet count, an enhanced risk of bleeding.

If the patient is receiving heparin therapy, monitor APTT results carefully because they may vary from test to test.

Alanine aminotransferase

One of two specialized enzymes called aminotransferases that can build up in the bloodstream when liver cells are injured, alanine aminotransferase (ALT) serves as an indicator of hepatic disease. Unlike aspartate aminotransferase (AST), the other aminotransferase, ALT appears primarily in the cytoplasm of liver cells, with smaller amounts in the kidneys, heart, and skeletal muscles. Because of this, ALT is a more specific indicator of acute liver cell damage than AST. After such damage, serum ALT levels may not return to normal for days or weeks.

You also may hear this test referred to as alanine transaminase or serum glutamic-pyruvic transaminase (SGPT).

Purpose
● To help detect and evaluate treatment of hepatic disease — especially hepatitis, and cirrhosis without jaundice
● To help distinguish between myocardial and hepatic tissue damage (when used with AST test)
● To assess hepatotoxicity of certain drugs.

Procedure-related nursing care
Explain the test's purpose to the patient and tell him you'll need to take a blood sample.

Perform a venipuncture, collecting the sample in a 7-ml red-top tube. If necessary, you can store the serum sample for up to 3 days at room temperature.

Reference values
In men, reference values range from 10 to 32 units/liter; in women, from 9 to 24 units/liter. The range for infants is twice that of adults.

Abnormal results
Extremely high levels of ALT (up to 50 times normal) suggest viral or severe drug-induced hepatitis, or another hepatic disease with extensive necrosis. (AST levels may also rise, but usually not as much.)

Moderate to high elevations may indicate infectious mononucleosis, chronic hepatitis, intrahepatic cholestasis or cholecystitis, early or improving acute viral hepatitis, or severe hepatic congestion caused by heart failure.

Slight to moderate elevations (usually with a greater increase in AST levels than in ALT levels) may appear in any condition that produces acute hepatocellular injury — such as active cirrhosis and drug-induced or alcoholic hepatitis. Marginal elevations occasionally occur in acute myocardial infarction, reflecting secondary hepatic congestion or the release of small amounts of ALT from myocardial tissue.

Nursing implications of abnormal results
If the patient has abnormally high ALT levels, watch for signs of jaundice. If you note such signs, provide good hygiene to help control odor and prevent skin breakdown, and try to relieve the patient's discomfort and itching.

Aldosterone, serum

This test measures serum levels of aldosterone, the principal mineralocorticoid secreted by the zona glomerulosa of the adrenal cortex. Aldosterone regulates ion transport across cell membranes in the renal tubules, helping to maintain blood pressure and volume and to regulate fluid and electrolyte balance.

Aldosterone secretion is controlled primarily by the renin-angiotensin system, serum potassium levels, and adrenocorticotropic hormone. As a result hyponatremia, hypovolemia, and other disorders that provoke renin release stimulate aldosterone secretion. Similarly, high potassium levels trigger aldosterone secretion through a potent feedback system.

This test is used to identify aldosteronism. When analyzed with plasma renin levels, the test results can help distinguish between the primary and secondary forms of this disorder. (For more information, see *Urine aldosterone test.*)

Purpose
• To help diagnose primary and secondary aldosteronism, hypoaldosteronism, and salt-losing syndrome.

Procedure-related nursing care
Explain the test's purpose to the patient, and tell him the test requires two blood samples. Instruct him to maintain a low-carbohydrate, normal-sodium (3 g/day or 135 μ/mol) diet for at least 2 weeks (preferably 30 days) before the test.

If the patient is premenopausal, specify the phase of her menstrual cycle on the laboratory slip. (Aldosterone levels may fluctuate during the menstrual cycle.) If aldosterone levels will be measured using radioimmunoassay, make sure the patient hasn't undergone a radioactive scan during the week preceding the test.

Perform a venipuncture in the morning while the patient is still supine after a night's rest. Collect the sample in a 7-ml red-top tube, and send it to the laboratory. On the slip, note the time and the patient's position during venipuncture.

Draw another sample 4 hours later with the patient standing, after he has been up and about. Use another 7-ml red-top collection tube, and send it to the laboratory. Note the time and the patient's position on the laboratory slip.

Tell the patient he can resume his normal diet.

Reference values
Reference values for a man or woman who has been supine for at least 2 hours are 7.4 ± 4.2 ng/dl (200 ± 11 pmol/L). Values for a man who has been upright for at least 4 hours are 5 to 30 ng/dl (0.14 to 0.83 nmol/L); for a woman who has been upright for at least 4 hours, 6 to 22 ng/dl (0.17 to 0.61 nmol/L).

Urine aldosterone test

Used to confirm a diagnosis of aldosteronism after serum tests show abnormal electrolyte and renin levels, this test requires a 24-hour urine specimen. Urine aldosterone levels closely reflect serum levels, but the urine test reflects the total daily secretion of aldosterone. Unlike the serum test results, the urine test results aren't affected by temporary fluctuations of aldosterone levels.

Procedure-related nursing care
Make sure the patient hasn't had a radioactive scan within the last week; it can interfere with the results.

Tell the patient to maintain a normal-sodium diet (3 g/day) before the test but to refrain from consuming sodium-rich foods such as bacon. Also tell him to avoid strenuous physical exercise and stressful situations during the collection period.

Collect a 24-hour urine specimen in a bottle containing a preservative. This will keep the specimen pH at 4.0 to 4.5. Refrigerate the specimen or keep it on ice during the collection period.

After you've collected a 24-hour specimen, send it to the laboratory immediately.

Reference values
Levels usually range from 2 to 16 μg/ 24 hours (5 to 45 nmol/d).

Abnormal results
Elevated levels suggest primary or secondary aldosteronism. Suppressed levels may result from Addison's disease, salt-losing syndrome, or toxemia of pregnancy.

Abnormal results
Excessive aldosterone secretion points to primary or secondary aldosteronism. Primary aldosteronism (Conn's syndrome) may result from adrenocortical adenoma, bilateral

adrenal hyperplasia or, less commonly, carcinoma. Secondary aldosteronism can result from conditions that increase renin-angiotensin activity, such as salt depletion, potassium excess, renovascular hypertension, congestive heart failure, cirrhosis, nephrotic syndrome, and idiopathic cyclic edema. Other causes include adrenocorticotropic hormone treatment and the third trimester of pregnancy.

Depressed aldosterone levels may indicate primary hypoaldosteronism, salt-losing syndrome, toxemia of pregnancy, Addison's disease, renin deficiency, or hypokalemia.

Nursing implications of abnormal results

Monitor the blood pressure of a patient with abnormal test results. An elevated blood pressure may indicate aldosteronism; a low blood pressure, hypoaldosteronism. Also carefully monitor the patient's serum electrolyte levels. In aldosteronism, hypokalemic alkalosis may occur, causing weakness, fatigue, areflexia, tetany, and arrhythmias. In hypoaldosteronism, hyperkalemia can lead to cardiac disturbances, even cardiac arrest.

Alkaline phosphatase

This test, which measures serum levels of alkaline phosphatase, serves as the primary indicator of space-occupying hepatic lesions. The reason: Alkaline phosphatase levels are particularly sensitive to mild biliary obstruction.

An enzyme that's most active at a pH of about 9.0, alkaline phosphatase influences bone calcification and lipid and metabolite transport.

Total serum levels reflect the combined activity of several alkaline phosphatase isoenzymes found in the liver, bones, kidneys, intestinal lining, and placenta.

Purpose
● To detect focal hepatic lesions causing biliary obstruction, such as tumors or abscesses
● To supplement information from other liver function studies and GI enzyme tests
● To detect skeletal diseases primarily characterized by marked osteoblastic activity
● To assess vitamin D therapy used for deficiency-induced rickets.

Procedure-related nursing care
Explain the purpose of the test to the patient, and tell him it requires a blood sample. Instruct him to fast for 10 to 12 hours before the test. Without the fast, fat intake will stimulate intestinal alkaline phosphatase secretion.

Perform a venipuncture, collecting the sample in a 7-ml red-top tube. Send it to the laboratory at once. If it remains at room temperature, alkaline phosphatase activity will increase because of a rise in the pH.

After the venipuncture, tell the patient to resume his normal diet.

Reference values
Benchmark serum alkaline phosphatase levels vary with the laboratory method used. Measured by the most common method, total alkaline phosphatase levels range from 30 to 120 units/liter in adults and from 40 to 200 units/liter in children. Because alkaline phosphatase concentrations rise during active bone formation and growth, infants, children, and adolescents may have levels up to three times as high as those of adults. Pregnancy also causes a

physiologic rise in alkaline phosphatase levels.

The reference range for the Bodansky method is 1.5 to 4 Bodansky units/dl; for the King-Armstrong method, 4 to 13.5 King-Armstrong units/dl; and for the Bessey-Lowry method, 0.8 to 2.5 Bessey-Lowry units/dl.

Abnormal results

Significant elevations in alkaline phosphatase levels usually indicate skeletal disease or an extrahepatic or intrahepatic biliary obstruction that causes cholestasis. Many acute hepatic diseases also cause alkaline phosphatase levels to rise before serum bilirubin levels change.

A moderate increase may reflect acute biliary obstruction from hepatocellular inflammation in active cirrhosis, mononucleosis, or viral hepatitis. Or such an increase may reflect osteomalacia or deficiency-induced rickets.

A sharp increase in alkaline phosphatase levels may indicate complete biliary obstruction by malignant or infectious infiltrations or fibrosis. Such markedly high levels are most common in Paget's disease and occur occasionally in biliary obstruction, extensive bone metastases, or hyperparathyroidism.

Rarely, low alkaline phosphatase levels can signal hypophosphatasia or protein or magnesium deficiency.

Nursing implications of abnormal results

If the test results and the patient's clinical picture suggest a hepatobiliary disorder, anticipate further liver function studies.

If the patient's increased alkaline phosphatase levels may stem from a skeletal or hepatic disease, you may need to prepare him for an isoenzyme fractionation test. He may also need other enzyme tests, such as serum gamma-glutamyltransferase, acid phosphatase, 5'-nucleotidase, and leucine aminopeptidase.

Ammonia, plasma

Used to help determine the severity of hepatocellular damage, this test measures plasma levels of ammonia — a nonprotein nitrogen compound that helps maintain acid-base balance. Most ammonia is absorbed from the intestinal tract, where it's produced by bacterial action on protein. The kidneys also produce a small amount from hydrolysis of glutamine.

Normally, the body uses the nitrogen fraction of ammonia to rebuild amino acids. The ammonia is then converted to urea in the liver for excretion by the kidneys. But in liver diseases, ammonia can bypass the liver and accumulate in the blood.

Purpose

• To help monitor the progression of severe hepatic disease and the effectiveness of therapy
• To recognize impending or established hepatic coma.

Procedure-related nursing care

If the patient is conscious, explain the purpose of the test and tell him it requires a blood sample. Tell him to fast overnight because protein intake may alter the test results.

Before performing the venipuncture, notify laboratory personnel so they can start their preparations. They'll have only 20 minutes from the time you draw the sample to perform the test.

Perform the venipuncture, collecting the sample in a 10-ml green-top tube. Handle the sample gently to prevent hemolysis. Pack the container in ice and send it to the laboratory immediately. (Don't use a chilled container.)

Before removing pressure from the venipuncture site, make sure the bleeding has stopped. Hepatic disease can prolong bleeding time.

Reference values
Plasma ammonia levels are normally less than 50 µg/dl (35 µmol/L).

Abnormal results
Severe hepatic disease and hepatic coma caused by cirrhosis or acute hepatic necrosis commonly cause elevated plasma ammonia levels. High levels also occur in Reye's syndrome, GI hemorrhage, severe congestive heart failure, pericarditis, erythroblastosis fetalis, and leukemia.

Nursing implications of abnormal results
Monitor a patient with high plasma ammonia levels for signs of hepatic coma. You may note slight personality changes, asterixis, confusion, lethargy, and stupor before the patient becomes comatose.

As ordered, provide a patient who has high plasma ammonia levels with a low-protein diet. This helps eliminate ammonia-producing material from the GI tract. Also provide catharsis to produce osmotic diarrhea and prevent ammonia-producing blood proteins and nitrogenous wastes from accumulating.

Neomycin and kanamycin may be ordered for this patient to suppress bacterial growth, which converts amino acids into ammonia. Lactulose may also be ordered to increase colonic acidity — another means of preventing bacterial growth — and to promote ammonia excretion. Occa-

sionally, hemodialysis or exchange transfusions may provide dramatic temporary relief.

Amylase, serum

When a doctor suspects acute pancreatic disease, he'll order either a serum or urine amylase measurement. An enzyme synthesized primarily in the pancreas and the salivary glands, and secreted into the GI tract, amylase helps digest starch and glycogen in the mouth, stomach, and intestines.

More than 20 methods of measuring serum amylase exist, with different ranges of reference values. Unfortunately, test values can't always be converted to a standard measurement. The classic saccharogenic method described here reports serum amylase in Somogyi units/dl.

Purpose
● To diagnose acute pancreatitis
● To distinguish acute pancreatitis from causes of abdominal pain that require immediate surgery
● To assess pancreatic injury caused by abdominal trauma or surgery.

Procedure-related nursing care
Explain the test's purpose to the patient, and tell him you'll need a blood sample. Instruct him to refrain from alcohol before the test.

Perform the venipuncture, collecting the sample in a 7-ml red-top tube. For the most accurate results, perform the venipuncture as soon as possible. The procedure should be done before other diagnostic or therapeutic interventions. If the patient reports severe pain in his left upper abdominal quadrant, collect the sample immediately.

Urine amylase test

When serum amylase levels are normal or borderline, this test can help diagnose acute pancreatitis. That's because serum amylase levels fall to normal within 3 days of the onset of acute pancreatitis, whereas urine amylase levels stay elevated for 7 to 10 days.

This test can also help diagnose chronic pancreatitis and salivary gland disorders.

Procedure-related nursing care
If the patient is menstruating, you may have to reschedule the test.

Collect the urine specimen over a 2-, 6-, 8-, or 24-hour period, as ordered. During the collection period, keep the specimen covered and refrigerated. For a catheterized patient, keep the collection bag on ice.

At the end of the collection period, send the specimen to the laboratory.

Reference values
Because laboratories report urine amylase in various units of measure, reported values differ. The Mayo Clinic reports excretion of 10 to 80 amylase units/hour (0 to 17 U/h) as normal.

Abnormal results
In response to most disorders, urine amylase levels rise and fall with serum amylase levels. However, in the later stages of acute pancreatitis, urine levels remain elevated after serum levels return to normal.

Reference values
Serum levels normally range from 60 to 180 Somogyi units/dl (40 to 130 U/L).

Abnormal results
The highest serum amylase levels occur 4 to 12 hours after the onset of acute pancreatitis. In 48 to 72 hours, the levels drop to normal. If the doctor suspects pancreatitis but the patient has normal serum levels, a urine test should be ordered. (For more information, see *Urine amylase test*.)

Moderate serum elevations may result from an obstruction of the common bile duct, the pancreatic duct, or the ampulla of Vater; pancreatic injury from a perforated peptic ulcer; pancreatic cancer; acute salivary gland disease; ectopic pregnancy; peritonitis; ovarian or lung cancer; and impaired renal function.

Slight elevations may occur in an asymptomatic patient. An amylase fractionation test may help determine the source of the amylase and aid in the selection of further tests.

Depressed levels can result from chronic pancreatitis, pancreatic cancer, cirrhosis, hepatitis, and toxemia of pregnancy.

Nursing implications of abnormal results
A serum amylase level above 200 Somogyi units/dl almost certainly indicates pancreatitis — especially if the patient also has elevated urine amylase and serum lipase levels. Observe this patient for other signs of pancreatitis and monitor his amylase levels. If his serum amylase levels drop but his urine amylase levels rise, the disorder's acute phase may be over. But if serum amylase levels remain elevated for more than 3 days, destruction of pancreatic tissue probably is continuing.

If elevated levels resulted from alcoholism, refer the patient for counseling.

Anion gap

The anion gap test measures the difference between serum levels of two anions, chloride (Cl^-) and bicarbonate (HCO_3^-), on the one hand and serum levels of two cations, sodium (Na^+) and potassium (K^+), on the other hand. The calculation of the anion gap is based on this physical principle: *Total* concentrations of cations and anions are normally equal, accounting for the electrical neutrality of serum. Thus, any gap between the measured anions and cations reflects the serum concentration of unmeasured anions: sulfates, phosphates, organic acids (such as ketone bodies and lactic acid), and proteins. (See *Functions of the major serum electrolytes*.)

An increased anion gap indicates a rise in one or more of these unmeasured anions. This may occur in acidosis characterized by excessive organic or inorganic acids, including lactic acidosis and ketoacidosis.

A normal anion gap, however, doesn't rule out metabolic acidosis. When acidosis results from a loss of HCO_3^- in the urine or other body fluids, renal reabsorption of Na^+ promotes Cl^- retention, and the anion gap remains unchanged. Thus, metabolic acidosis resulting from excessive Cl^- levels is known as normal anion gap acidosis.

The hypokalemic form of normal anion gap acidosis results from renal tubular acidosis, diarrhea, or ureteral diversions. The hyperkalemic form can stem from acidifying agents (for example, ammonium chloride and hydrochloric acid) and renal disorders such as hydrone-

Functions of the major serum electrolytes

ION	ELECTROLYTE	FUNCTIONS
Cations		
	Sodium (Na^+)	• Maintains osmotic pressure of extracellular fluid • Helps regulate neuromuscular activity • Influences acid-base balance and chloride and potassium levels • Helps regulate water excretion
	Potassium (K^+)	• Maintains cellular osmotic equilibrium • Helps regulate neuromuscular and enzymatic activity and acid-base balance • Influences kidney function
Anions		
	Chloride (Cl^-)	• Influences acid-base balance • Helps maintain blood osmotic pressure and arterial pressure
	Bicarbonate (HCO_3^-)	• Acts with carbonic acid in buffer system that regulates blood pH

phrosis, amyloidosis, nephritis, and sickle cell nephropathy.

Purpose
• To distinguish types of metabolic acidosis
• To monitor renal function in a patient receiving total parenteral nutrition.

Procedure-related nursing care
Explain the test's purpose to the patient, and tell him the test requires a blood sample. Then perform a venipuncture and collect the sample in a 10- to 15-ml red-top tube.

Reference values
The anion gap should range from 8 to 14 mEq/liter (mmol/L).

Abnormal results
An anion gap above 14 mEq/liter results from the buildup of metabolic acids and occurs with conditions that cause organic acids, sulfates, or phosphates to accumulate. Such conditions include renal failure; ketoacidosis from starvation, diabetes mellitus, or alcohol ingestion; lactic acidosis; and salicylate, methanol, ethylene glycol (antifreeze), or paraldehyde toxicity.

Although rare, an anion gap below 8 mEq/liter may occur in hypermagnesemia and in paraproteinemic states, such as multiple myeloma and Waldenström's macroglobulinemia.

Nursing implications of abnormal results
If the patient has an increased anion gap, he may need further tests to determine the specific cause of his metabolic acidosis. Monitor this patient for such signs and symptoms as Kussmaul's respirations, increased pulse rate, flushed skin, fruity breath odor, lethargy, and

drowsiness progressing to coma.

Monitor his arterial blood gas and serum electrolyte levels. Metabolic acidosis results in decreased pH and HCO_3^- levels. If respiratory compensation occurs, partial pressure of carbon dioxide in arterial blood will also decrease. Serum potassium levels typically rise.

As ordered, treat the patient for metabolic acidosis. Treatment will vary, although it usually includes sodium bicarbonate administration.

Arterial blood gas analysis

Arterial blood gas (ABG) analysis evaluates gas exchange in the lungs by measuring the partial pressures of oxygen (PaO_2) and carbon dioxide ($PaCO_2$) in arterial blood. PaO_2 indicates how much oxygen the lungs are delivering to the blood. $PaCO_2$ indicates how efficiently the lungs eliminate carbon dioxide.

The test also measures the arterial sample's pH, which indicates the acid-base balance, or the hydrogen ion (H^+) concentration. Acidity indicates an H^+ excess; alkalinity, an H^+ deficit. Other ABG measurements include oxygen (O_2) content, oxygen saturation (SaO_2), and bicarbonate (HCO_3^-) levels. (See *ABG glossary,* page 20.)

You may draw blood for ABG analysis by percutaneous arterial puncture or from an arterial line.

Purpose
• To evaluate the efficiency of pulmonary gas exchange
• To determine the blood's acid-base balance
• To monitor respiratory therapy
• To assess the efficiency of mechanical ventilation.

ABG glossary

☐ Acidosis: A loss of base or an accumulation of acid resulting from metabolic or respiratory changes.
☐ Alkalosis: A loss of acid or an accumulation of base resulting from metabolic or respiratory changes.
☐ O_2 content: Oxygen content.
☐ Partial pressure: A measure of the force that a gas exerts on the fluid in which it's dissolved.
☐ $PaCO_2$: Partial pressure of carbon dioxide in arterial blood.
☐ PaO_2: Partial pressure of oxygen in arterial blood.
☐ pH: A measure of acid-base balance or the concentration of free hydrogen ions in the blood.
☐ SaO_2: Oxygen saturation, a percentage indicating the amount of oxygen combined with hemoglobin compared to the total oxygen that could be combined with hemoglobin.

Procedure-related nursing care

Take the following actions before, during, and after the procedure.

Before the procedure. Explain the test to the patient, and tell him it requires a blood sample. Instruct him to breathe normally while you draw the sample. If you need to perform an arterial puncture, warn him that he may feel a brief cramping or throbbing pain at the puncture site.

If the patient has just started receiving mechanical ventilation, wait at least 15 minutes before drawing the sample. That way, you'll get an accurate measurement of the patient's response to mechanical ventilation. If a patient is receiving oxygen therapy, discontinue it for 15 to 20 minutes, if ordered, before drawing a sample. With a patient receiving intermittent positive-pressure breathing, wait at least 20 minutes after treatment stops before drawing the sample; such treatment alters ABG values. For the same reason, don't suction a patient right before drawing an arterial sample.

During the procedure. Perform an arterial puncture or collect the sample from the arterial line, drawing the blood into a heparinized syringe. Put the sample into a bag of ice.

After the procedure. If you performed an arterial puncture, apply pressure to the puncture site for at least 5 minutes — 10 minutes if you used the femoral artery — and tape a gauze pad firmly over it. Avoid taping around the entire limb.

Note on the requisition slip whether the patient was receiving oxygen therapy or breathing room air when you drew the sample. If appropriate, note the oxygen flow rate. For a patient receiving mechanical ventilation, note the fraction of inspired oxygen (FIO_2) and tidal volume. For any patient, note the rectal temperature and respiratory rate. Send the sample and the requisition slip to the laboratory.

Monitor the patient's vital signs. Observe a patient who received an arterial puncture for signs and symptoms of circulatory impairment, including swelling, discoloration, pain, numbness, and tingling in the bandaged arm or leg, and check the puncture site for bleeding.

Reference values

ABG values should fall within these ranges:
- O_2 content: 15% to 23%
- PaO_2: 75 to 100 mm Hg
- $PaCO_2$: 35 to 45 mm Hg
- pH: 7.35 to 7.42
- SaO_2: 94% to 100%
- HCO_3^-: 22 to 26 mEq/liter.

Recognizing acid-base disorders

DISORDER	A.B.G. FINDINGS	POSSIBLE CAUSES
Respiratory acidosis (excess CO_2 retention)	• pH < 7.35 • HCO_3^- > 26 mEq/liter (if compensating) • $PaCO_2$ > 45 mm Hg	• Central nervous system depression from drugs, injury, or disease • Hypoventilation from respiratory, cardiac, musculoskeletal, or neuromuscular disease
Respiratory alkalosis (excess CO_2 loss)	• pH > 7.42 • HCO_3^- < 22 mEq/liter (if compensating) • $PaCO_2$ < 35 mm Hg	• Hyperventilation due to anxiety, pain, or improper ventilator settings • Respiratory stimulation from drugs, disease, hypoxia, fever, or high room temperature • Gram-negative bacteremia
Metabolic acidosis (HCO_3^- loss or acid retention)	• pH < 7.35 • HCO_3^- < 22 mEq/liter • $PaCO_2$ < 35 mm Hg (if compensating)	• Depletion of HCO_3^- from renal disease, diarrhea, or small-bowel fistulas • Excessive production of organic acids from hepatic disease; endocrine disorders, such as diabetes mellitus; hypoxia; shock; or drug toxicity • Inadequate excretion of acids due to renal disease
Metabolic alkalosis (HCO_3^- retention or acid loss)	• pH > 7.42 • HCO_3^- > 26 mEq/liter • $PaCO_2$ > 45 mm Hg (if compensating)	• Loss of hydrochloric acid from prolonged vomiting or gastric suctioning • Loss of potassium from increased renal excretion (as in diuretic therapy) or steroid overdose • Excessive alkali ingestion

Abnormal results

A PaO_2 level below 50 mm Hg in an adult usually indicates hypoxia; however, in a neonate, 40 to 60 mm Hg may be normal. A value below 80 mm Hg may indicate hypoxia, depending on the patient's age and the oxygen concentration he's receiving. After age 60, a patient's normal PaO_2 may fall below 80 mm Hg.

A $PaCO_2$ above 45 mm Hg indicates hypoventilation, or hypercapnia. A level below 35 mm Hg signals hyperventilation, or hypocapnia. The $PaCO_2$ value can also signal a respiratory acid-base imbalance. A level above 45 mm Hg points to respiratory acidosis; below 35 mm Hg, respiratory alkalosis.

A pH greater than 7.42 indicates alkalosis. A pH less than 7.35 indicates acidosis.

A patient with a PaO_2 between 60 and 100 mm Hg should have an SaO_2 above 85%. If his SaO_2 drops sharply, his PaO_2 has probably fallen below 50 mm Hg.

An HCO_3^- value above 26 mEq/liter points to metabolic, or kidney-related, alkalosis; under 22 mEq/liter, metabolic acidosis. (For more information, see *Recognizing acid-base disorders.*)

Nursing implications of abnormal results

If the patient's ABG values reveal hypoxemia, tell the doctor at once. Initiate or adjust oxygen therapy, as ordered.

Monitor the patient with abnormal

ABG values for signs of acid-base disturbances. Signs may include a decreased level of consciousness, possibly progressing to coma, and arrhythmias from an electrolyte imbalance. Each type of acid-base disturbance also has its own characteristic signs and symptoms.

• *Metabolic acidosis.* Look for lethargy, weakness, drowsiness, anorexia, nausea and vomiting, abdominal pain, and flushing. Respiratory compensation may also lead to Kussmaul's respirations.

• *Metabolic alkalosis.* Observe the patient for dizziness, paresthesia in the hands and face, muscle spasms, seizures, anorexia, and nausea and vomiting. A fluid and electrolyte imbalance may also lead to diarrhea; respiratory compensation can produce shallow breathing.

• *Respiratory acidosis.* This can cause a headache, drowsiness, and decreased respiratory rate and depth.

• *Respiratory alkalosis.* Monitor the patient for signs of dizziness, paresthesia, muscle weakness and spasm, and tachypnea.

If the patient's ABG values and signs and symptoms indicate a specific acid-base disturbance, treat the complications as ordered. Take measures to help him breathe normally and to reverse any fluid or electrolyte abnormalities. Teach him about the cause and management of the underlying disorder.

Aspartate aminotransferase

Aspartate aminotransferase (AST) serves as an indicator of hepatic and cardiac diseases. A hepatic enzyme,

AST is found in the cytoplasm and mitochondria of many cells — mainly in the liver, heart, skeletal muscles, kidneys, pancreas and, to a lesser extent, the red blood cells (RBCs). When cellular damage occurs, AST is released into serum.

Even though a correlation exists between high AST levels and myocardial infarction (MI), some clinicians consider this test alone inconclusive for diagnosing an MI. That's because the test can't differentiate between acute MI and hepatic congestion from heart failure.

You also may hear this test referred to as aspartate transaminase or serum glutamic-oxaloacetic transaminase (SGOT).

Purpose
• To aid in the detection and differential diagnosis of acute hepatic disease
• To monitor progress in patients with cardiac or hepatic diseases
• To detect a recent MI (together with creatine phosphokinase and lactate dehydrogenase tests).

Procedure-related nursing care
Explain the test's purpose to the patient. Tell him the test usually requires three venipunctures — one on admission and one each day for the next 2 days.

Perform the venipuncture, collecting the sample in a 7-ml red-top tube. To obtain the most reliable results, draw serum samples at the same time each day.

Reference values
AST levels should range from 8 to 20 units/liter. For infants, levels can be as much as four times those for adults.

Abnormal results
AST levels fluctuate according to

the extent of cellular necrosis. Thus, levels may rise slightly and transiently early in the disorder and peak during the most acute phase. Depending on when the initial sample is drawn, subsequent AST levels may rise — indicating increasing tissue damage — or fall — indicating tissue repair. These relative changes provide a reliable way to monitor cellular damage.

Extremely high elevations (more than 20 times normal) may indicate acute viral hepatitis, severe skeletal muscle trauma, extensive surgery, drug-induced hepatic injury, or severe passive hepatic congestion.

High elevations (from 10 to 20 times normal) can result from severe MI, severe infectious mononucleosis, and alcoholic cirrhosis. Such levels may also occur during the prodromal or resolution stages of conditions that cause extremely high elevations.

Moderate to high elevations (from 5 to 10 times normal) may point to Duchenne's muscular dystrophy, dermatomyositis, or chronic hepatitis. These levels can also occur during the prodromal and resolution stages of diseases that cause high elevations.

Low to moderate elevations (from 2 to 5 times normal) may indicate hemolytic anemia, metastatic hepatic tumors, acute pancreatitis, pulmonary emboli, alcohol withdrawal syndrome, or fatty liver.

AST levels rise slightly after the first few days of a biliary duct obstruction. Relatively low elevations also occur at some time during all of the preceding conditions.

Nursing implications of abnormal results

If the patient has an elevated AST level, carefully assess him to help determine the cause. If liver damage may have caused high AST levels, check the results of liver function studies.

If MI is suspected, you'll probably check for elevations of other serum enzyme levels — especially creatine phosphokinase (CPK) and lactate dehydrogenase (LDH) isoenzymes — that are more definitive indicators of MI. Monitor the AST levels of a patient diagnosed with MI. A rise to more than five times normal or a prolonged elevation may signal a poor prognosis.

Bilirubin, serum

This test measures serum levels of bilirubin, the predominant pigment in bile. The major product of hemoglobin catabolism, bilirubin is formed in the reticuloendothelial system. Bilirubin is then bound to albumin, a plasma protein, and transported to the liver as unconjugated (indirect or prehepatic) bilirubin. There it joins with glucuronic acid to form bilirubin glucuronide and bilirubin diglucuronide, and is excreted into bile as conjugated (direct or posthepatic) bilirubin.

Effective bilirubin conjugation and excretion depend on a properly functioning hepatobiliary system and a normal turnover rate of red blood cells (RBCs). Thus, measuring levels of indirect and direct bilirubin can help evaluate hepatobiliary function and RBC production. Urine bilirubin levels can help confirm a diagnosis. (See *Urine bilirubin test*, page 24.)

Serum bilirubin measurements are particularly significant in neonates because indirect bilirubin can accumulate in the brain, causing irreparable tissue damage.

Urine bilirubin test

When a patient has jaundice, this test can help identify the cause, although results must be correlated with serum bilirubin and urine and fecal urobilinogen levels. The test uses a color reaction to a reagent to detect abnormally high urine concentrations of direct bilirubin.

Procedure-related nursing care
Collect a random urine specimen in the appropriate container. Immediately test the specimen or send it to the laboratory. Bilirubin disintegrates after only 30 minutes of exposure to room temperature or light. If you'll be testing the specimen at bedside, be sure you have adequate lighting.

For bedside analysis, you may use one of these procedures:
• Dipstrip. Dip the reagent strip into the specimen and remove it immediately. After 20 seconds, compare the strip color with the color standards.
• Icotest. This test is more sensitive than the Dipstrip. Place five drops of urine on the asbestos cellulose test mat. The mat will absorb any bilirubin in the urine. Next, put a reagent tablet on the wet area of the mat and place two drops of water on the tablet. A blue to purple coloration will develop on the mat if it has absorbed any bilirubin. Pink or red indicates an absence of bilirubin.

With either method, record the test results on the patient's chart.

If the specimen will be analyzed in the laboratory, record the collection time on the patient's chart. If hepatitis is suspected, attach the appropriate biohazard label to the container.

Normal results
Bilirubin isn't normally found in urine.

Abnormal results
Bilirubin in the urine may indicate extrahepatic obstruction, hepatocellular disorders (such as hepatitis and cirrhosis), or hepatocanalicular disorders or intrahepatic obstruction (such as drug-induced cholestasis and primary biliary cirrhosis).

Purpose
• To evaluate liver function
• To help detect jaundice and monitor its progression
• To help diagnose biliary obstruction and hemolytic anemia
• To determine whether a neonate needs treatment for dangerously high levels of indirect bilirubin.

Procedure-related nursing care
Explain the test's purpose to the patient—or to his parents if the patient is a neonate. Tell an adult patient to fast for at least 4 hours before the test. (A neonate doesn't need to fast.)

Explain that the test requires a blood sample. Tell a neonate's parents that you'll need to draw a small amount of blood from the infant's heel.

With an adult patient, perform a venipuncture, collecting the sample in a 10- to 15-ml red-top tube. With a neonate, perform a heel stick and collect the blood in a microcapillary tube.

Once you've collected the sample, protect it from strong sunlight and ultraviolet light. Remember, bilirubin breaks down when exposed to light.

Tell an adult patient that he may resume his normal diet.

Reference values
Indirect serum bilirubin should measure at or below 1.1 mg/dl (18 µmol/L); direct serum bilirubin, less

than 0.5 mg/dl (8 μmol/L). Total serum bilirubin levels in neonates range from 1 to 12 mg/dl (17 to 205 μmol/L).

Abnormal results

Elevated indirect serum bilirubin levels can result from hemolysis, transfusion reaction, hemolytic or pernicious anemia, hemorrhage, hepatocellular dysfunction (possibly resulting from viral hepatitis or congenital enzyme deficiencies, such as Gilbert's syndrome and Crigler-Najjar syndrome), and neonatal hepatic immaturity.

Elevated direct serum bilirubin levels usually indicate biliary obstruction. In this disorder, direct bilirubin, blocked from its normal pathway through the liver into the biliary tree, overflows into the bloodstream. Such obstruction may be intrahepatic (from viral hepatitis, cirrhosis, or a chlorpromazine reaction) or extrahepatic (from gallstones or gallbladder or pancreatic carcinoma). An obstruction also may result from bile duct disease.

If the biliary obstruction continues, indirect bilirubin levels may also rise because of hepatic damage. In severe chronic hepatic damage, direct bilirubin levels may return to normal or near-normal levels eventually, but indirect bilirubin levels remain elevated.

In a neonate, a total bilirubin level of 20 mg/dl (340 μmol/L) or more indicates the need for an exchange transfusion.

Nursing implications of abnormal results

Observe any patient who has an elevated bilirubin level for signs of jaundice, including yellow sclera, yellowish skin, dark-colored urine, and light stools. If the patient has jaundice, give him an antipruritic

drug as ordered and rub oil-based lotions on his skin to relieve pruritus and prevent skin breakdown.

If a neonate has a total bilirubin level of 20 mg/dl or more, prepare him for an exchange transfusion.

Keep in mind that 50% of all neonates have physiologic jaundice, which elevates the bilirubin level during the first few days of life. But usually, the level remains below 20 mg/dl. If a neonate has a bilirubin level above 20 mg/dl the first day, or if the level doesn't start to drop after 3 to 5 days, suspect pathologic jaundice.

A neonate's indirect bilirubin level also may rise because of lowered serum albumin levels, hypoxia, cold, stress, use of certain drugs, and other metabolic factors.

Blood urea nitrogen

Used to evaluate renal function, this test measures the nitrogen fraction of urea, the chief end product of protein metabolism. Formed in the liver from ammonia and excreted by the kidneys, urea accounts for 40% to 50% of the blood's nonprotein nitrogen.

The blood urea nitrogen (BUN) level reflects protein intake and renal excretory capacity. But the serum creatinine test is a more reliable indicator of uremia.

Purpose
• To evaluate renal function and aid in the diagnosis of renal disease
• To help assess hydration.

Procedure-related nursing care
Explain the test's purpose to the patient, and tell him you'll need a blood sample.

Perform a venipuncture, collecting the sample in a 10- to 15-ml red-top tube.

Reference values
BUN levels should range from 8 to 20 mg/dl (3 to 7.1 mmol/L).

Abnormal results
Elevated BUN levels occur in renal disease, reduced renal blood flow (caused by dehydration, for example), urinary tract obstruction, and conditions that increase protein catabolism (such as burns).

Depressed BUN levels occur in severe hepatic damage, malnutrition, and overhydration.

Nursing implications of abnormal results
When a patient has an elevated BUN level, check the results of his serum creatinine test. If those levels are also high, suspect impaired renal function. Monitor the patient's level of consciousness carefully. Impaired renal function can lead to a buildup of nitrogenous compounds in the blood, resulting in confusion and disorientation.

Monitor the fluid intake and urine output of any patient with an elevated BUN level. Report a urine output of less than 30 ml/hour.

BUN level elevations may cause seizures, so take the appropriate precautions. You'll also need to teach the patient and his family how to modify his diet to restrict protein intake.

Calcium, serum

Used to detect several disorders, this test measures serum levels of calcium—a cation that helps regulate and promote neuromuscular and enzyme activity, skeletal development, and blood coagulation. The body absorbs calcium from the GI tract, provided it contains sufficient vitamin D, and excretes calcium in the urine and feces. Over 98% of the body's calcium is found in the bones and teeth. But calcium can shift in and out of these structures. For example, when calcium concentrations in the blood drop below normal, calcium can move out of the bones and teeth to help restore blood levels.

Besides vitamin D, parathyroid hormone and, to a lesser extent, calcitonin and adrenal steroids also help control calcium blood levels (see *Understanding calcium absorption*). Calcium and phosphorus are closely related, usually reacting together to form insoluble calcium phosphate. To prevent this compound from precipitating in the blood, calcium levels vary inversely with phosphorus levels. As serum calcium levels rise, phosphorus levels should fall through renal excretion. Because the body excretes calcium, the diet must contain at least 1 g/day to maintain a normal calcium balance. (See also *Urine calcium test*, page 28.)

Purpose
• To help diagnose neuromuscular, skeletal, and endocrine disorders; arrhythmias; blood-clotting deficiencies; and acid-base imbalance.

Procedure-related nursing care
Explain the purpose of the test to the patient, and tell him it requires a blood sample. Then perform a venipuncture, collecting the sample in a 10- to 15-ml red-top tube.

Reference values
Serum calcium levels should range

Understanding calcium absorption

Because most calcium compounds are insoluble, they're poorly absorbed from the intestinal tract. Vitamin D_3 and parathyroid hormone play an important role in the intestinal absorption of calcium.

Calcium ingestion

In the presence of parathyroid hormone, the kidneys convert 25-hydroxycholecalciferol to 1,25-dihydroxycholecalciferol (the most active derivative of vitamin D_3). This conversion is necessary for calcium absorption from the small intestine.

Calcium passes through the stomach into the small intestine (duodenum), where absorption takes place. In the intestinal epithelium, 1,25-dihydroxycholecalciferol from the kidneys forms calcium-binding protein, calcium-stimulated ATPase, and alkaline phosphatase, which promote intestinal calcium absorption into the plasma.

When calcium-bearing plasma passes through the parathyroid glands, the calcium-ion concentration is identified. Based on the plasma calcium-ion concentration, parathyroid hormone is secreted into the bloodstream and travels to the kidneys. The higher the calcium-ion concentration, the less parathyroid hormone secreted; the lower the concentration, the more hormone secreted.

Once calcium ions pass into the plasma, they're absorbed by the bone, heart muscle, and nervous system cells as the plasma circulates throughout the body.

Urine calcium test

To evaluate calcium metabolism and excretion or to monitor treatment for a calcium deficiency, a patient's doctor may order a urine calcium test, requiring a 24-hour urine specimen.

Procedure-related nursing care
Encourage the patient to be as active as possible before the procedure. As ordered, make sure he follows the Albright-Reifenstein diet (which contains about 130 mg of calcium/day) for 3 days before the test.

Collect a 24-hour urine specimen and send it to the laboratory.

Reference values
Although levels vary with dietary intake, men normally excrete less than 275 mg/day (7 mmol/d); women, less than 250 mg/day (6 mmol/d).

Abnormal results
In response to most disorders, urine calcium levels increase or decrease along with serum levels. But if a disorder affects the kidneys, urine and serum calcium levels can differ significantly. In renal tubular acidosis, for instance, urine levels rise above serum levels; in renal failure, they drop below serum levels.

from 8.9 to 10.1 mg/dl (2.25 to 2.75 mmol/L). Children have higher serum calcium levels than adults. During phases of rapid bone growth, calcium levels can rise as high as 12 mg/dl (3 mmol/L).

Abnormal results
Abnormally high serum calcium levels (hypercalcemia) may occur in hyperparathyroidism and parathyroid tumors (caused by oversecretion of parathyroid hormone), Paget's disease of the bone, multiple myeloma, metastatic carcinoma, multiple fractures, or prolonged immobilization. Elevated serum calcium levels may also result from inadequate excretion of calcium, as in adrenal insufficiency and renal disease; excessive calcium ingestion; or overuse of antacids such as calcium carbonate.

Low calcium levels (hypocalcemia) may result from hypoparathyroidism, total parathyroidectomy, malabsorption, Cushing's syndrome, renal failure, acute pancreatitis, and peritonitis.

Nursing implications of abnormal results
Your actions will vary according to the test results.

Elevated serum calcium levels. Assess the patient with high serum calcium levels for symptoms of hypercalcemia, including deep bone pain, muscle hypotonicity, lethargy, and weakness. Be alert for a hypercalcemic crisis, which begins with nausea and vomiting, thirst, abdominal pain, anorexia, and dyspnea and can progress to stupor, coma, and cardiac arrest. Report signs and symptoms of hypercalcemic crisis at once.

If the patient's calcium level surpasses 14 mg/dl (or if it reaches 12 mg/dl and he has symptoms of hypercalcemia), provide immediate treatment. Administer I.V. fluids, as ordered, to promote calcium excretion in the urine. Usually, you'll give a diuretic as ordered (but not a thiazide) to foster urine formation and excretion and to prevent fluid overload. The patient will also need to receive magnesium and potassium supplements to prevent depletion. Once diuresis has begun, give him an antihypercalcemic agent, such as plicamycin or calcitonin, as ordered. The doctor may order inorganic phosphate as well.

Tell the patient to limit his calcium intake, as ordered. He'll also need to drink six to eight glasses of fluid each day, unless contraindicated, and to walk as much as possible to prevent calcium loss from the bone. If the patient is bedridden, help him with passive range-of-motion exercises.

Monitor a patient receiving digitalis for signs of toxicity, including nausea, vomiting, and arrhythmias such as bradycardia.

Decreased serum calcium levels. Assess the patient with low serum calcium levels for signs and symptoms of hypocalcemia, including circumoral and peripheral numbness and tingling, muscle twitching, Chvostek's sign (facial muscle spasm), tetany, muscle cramping, Trousseau's sign (carpopedal spasm), seizures, and arrhythmias. Report these signs and symptoms as soon as possible.

Provide immediate treatment for the patient with tetany. As ordered, administer I.V. calcium gluconate to increase serum calcium levels. Monitor his cardiac function to detect arrhythmias, and keep a tracheostomy tray and an endotracheal tube close by in case tetany causes an airway obstruction.

Remember, when serum calcium levels fall rapidly, neuromuscular symptoms may begin at levels only slightly below normal. If levels fall slowly, however, symptoms may not begin until calcium levels drop to 6 mg/dl.

Tell the patient to use antacids and laxatives as little as possible because they can lower serum calcium levels. Also, teach him to eat foods high in calcium and low in phosphorus and to take vitamin D and oral calcium supplements as prescribed.

Monitor a patient receiving digitalis and calcium supplements for signs of toxicity — including nausea, vomiting, and arrhythmias such as bradycardia — which may develop if calcium levels rise rapidly.

Chloride, serum

This test measures serum levels of chloride, the major extracellular fluid anion. Interacting with sodium, the major extracellular cation, chloride helps regulate blood volume and arterial pressure by helping maintain the osmotic pressure of blood.

Chloride levels affect acid-base balance, varying inversely with bicarbonate levels. Excessive chloride loss in gastric juices or other secretions can cause hypochloremic metabolic alkalosis; excessive chloride retention or ingestion can lead to hyperchloremic metabolic acidosis.

Absorbed from the intestines and excreted primarily by the kidneys, chloride can also be measured in urine. (See *Urine chloride test,* page 30.)

Purpose
● To detect acid-base imbalance
● To help evaluate fluid status and extracellular cation-anion balance.

Procedure-related nursing care
Explain the purpose of the test to the patient, and tell him it requires a blood sample. Perform a venipuncture, collecting the sample in a 10- to 15-ml red-top tube.

Reference values
Serum chloride levels should range from 100 to 108 mEq/liter (100 to 108 mmol/L).

Urine chloride test

Urine chloride measurements help you evaluate renal conservation of chloride and confirm serum values. To evaluate fluid and electrolyte imbalance, you must correlate urine chloride levels with the results of serum electrolyte studies.

Procedure-related nursing care
Tell the patient that the test requires a 24-hour urine specimen and, if necessary, teach him how to collect the sample. Make sure he understands that he must collect all his urine during the 24-hour period.

Reference values
Although levels vary greatly with salt intake and perspiration, normal urine chloride excretion usually ranges from 110 to 250 mEq/day.

Abnormal results
Elevated levels may result from dehydration, salicylate toxicity, diabetic acidosis, adrenocortical insufficiency (Addison's disease), and salt-losing renal disease. Diminished levels can stem from excessive diaphoresis, congestive heart failure, renal failure, and hypochloremic metabolic alkalosis after prolonged vomiting or gastric suctioning.

Abnormal results
Elevated chloride levels (hyperchloremia) can result from severe dehydration, complete renal shutdown, head injury (producing neurogenic hyperventilation), and primary aldosteronism.

Usually associated with low sodium and potassium levels, low chloride levels (hypochloremia) can stem from prolonged vomiting, gastric suctioning, intestinal fistula, chronic renal failure, and Addison's disease. Dilutional hypochloremia can result from congestive heart failure or edema that leads to excess extracellular fluid.

Nursing implications of abnormal results
Your actions will vary according to the test results.

Elevated serum chloride levels. Assess the patient with high serum chloride levels for signs and symptoms of hyperchloremia, including weakness, tachypnea, and rapid deep breathing. If unchecked, hyperchloremia may produce stupor and coma. Monitor the patient, too, for signs and symptoms of overhydration, which may accompany high chloride and sodium levels. These include weight gain, venous distention, dyspnea, cough, and crackles. Monitor the patient's fluid intake and output. Weigh him daily to check for fluid retention.

Teach him how to maintain a salt-restricted diet, as ordered. Make sure he knows he should check the labels of salt substitutes because some contain chloride.

Decreased serum chloride levels. Assess the patient with low serum chloride levels for signs and symptoms of hypochloremia, such as muscle hypertonicity, tetany, decreased respirations, and decreased blood pressure. Also monitor his serum sodium and potassium levels. A decrease in these electrolyte levels commonly signals a concomitant loss of chloride.

Assess the patient's fluid and electrolyte replacement therapy. Make sure he's receiving both potassium and chloride to correct hypokalemic-hypochloremic alkalosis, or the alkalosis will persist.

As ordered, set up an I.V. infusion of normal saline solution to replace lost electrolytes. Monitor the patient receiving a high volume for signs and symptoms of overhydration.

Teach the patient to increase his dietary chloride intake by including such foods as salt, broth, meat, seafood, and tomato juice in his diet.

Cholesterol, total

Used primarily to determine the risk of coronary artery disease (CAD), this test measures the circulating levels of free cholesterol and cholesterol esters—the two forms in which this biochemical compound appears in the body.

Cholesterol, a structural component in cell membranes and plasma lipoproteins, is absorbed from the diet and synthesized in the liver and other body tissues. It helps form adrenocorticoid steroids, bile salts, androgens, and estrogens.

A diet high in saturated fat raises cholesterol levels by stimulating the absorption of lipids, including cholesterol, from the intestine; a diet low in saturated fat lowers cholesterol levels.

Purpose
• To assess the risk of CAD
• To evaluate fat metabolism
• To help diagnose nephrotic syndrome, pancreatitis, hepatic disease, hypothyroidism, and hyperthyroidism.

Procedure-related nursing care
Explain the purpose of the test to the patient, and tell him it requires a blood sample. Make sure he fasts overnight and refrains from drinking alcohol for 24 hours before the procedure.

Perform a venipuncture, collecting the sample in a 7-ml red-top tube. Send it to the laboratory immediately; cholesterol isn't stable at room temperature.

After the procedure, tell the patient he may resume his normal diet.

Reference values
Total cholesterol concentrations vary with age and sex, normally ranging from 150 to 200 mg/dl (3.87 to 5.17 mmol/L).

Abnormal results
Cholesterol levels above 250 mg/dl generally indicate a high risk of CAD and the need for treatment. A patient with a level between 200 and 240 mg/dl has a moderate risk. But if he has other risk factors—if he smokes or has high blood pressure, for instance—his risk of CAD is considered high. Elevated cholesterol levels (hypercholesterolemia) can also indicate incipient hepatitis, lipid disorders, bile duct blockage, nephrotic syndrome, obstructive jaundice, pancreatitis, and hypothyroidism.

Low serum cholesterol levels (hypocholesterolemia) result from malnutrition, cellular necrosis of the liver, and hyperthyroidism.

Nursing implications of abnormal results
Abnormal results commonly call for further testing to pinpoint the disorder. A patient with suspected cardiovascular disease, for instance, may need a lipoprotein-cholesterol fractionation test.

If a patient has a high cholesterol level, teach him how to reduce it. Steps he can take include following a low-cholesterol diet, exercising and, if prescribed, taking medications that inhibit cholesterol absorption.

Creatine phosphokinase

An enzyme found mainly in muscle cells and brain tissue, creatine phosphokinase (CPK) — also known as creatine kinase — catalyzes the transfer of a phosphate group from adenosine triphosphate to creatine, releasing energy in the process. Because of this key role in energy production, CPK reflects tissue catabolism. An increase in serum CPK levels serves as an indicator of cellular trauma.

CPK occurs as three distinct isoenzymes: CPK-BB, found mainly in brain tissue; CPK-MB, located in cardiac muscle (although a small amount also appears in skeletal muscle); and CPK-MM, found in skeletal muscle. Because each isoenzyme is associated with a specific location, fractionation and measurement can help pinpoint the site of tissue destruction. Total CPK levels help diagnose skeletal muscle disorders, but CPK-MM, which constitutes over 99% of the total CPK normally present in serum, acts as a more specific indicator.

Purpose
• To diagnose acute myocardial infarction (MI) and reinfarction
• To evaluate possible causes of chest pain and to monitor the severity of myocardial ischemia after cardiac surgery or catheterization or cardioversion
• To detect skeletal muscle disorders that don't have a neurogenic origin, such as Duchenne muscular dystrophy and early dermatomyositis.

Procedure-related nursing care
Explain the test's purpose to the patient, and tell him you'll need to collect several blood samples. If he's being tested for a skeletal muscle disorder, instruct him to avoid exercising for 24 hours before the test.

Perform a venipuncture, collecting the sample in a 7-ml red-top tube. If the patient needs an I.M. injection, be sure to draw the sample either before the injection or at least 1 hour after it. Otherwise, the test results may be altered. Send the sample to the laboratory at once; CPK activity diminishes significantly after a sample is exposed to room temperature for 2 hours.

Always collect the sample on schedule, and note the time on the laboratory slip. For a patient with chest pain, note how many hours have elapsed since the pain started.

Reference values
Total CPK levels determined by the most commonly performed assay in North America range from 40 to 175 units/liter for men and from 25 to 140 units/liter for women. Typical ranges for isoenzyme levels are as follows: CPK-BB, undetectable; CPK-MB, undetectable to 7 units/liter; CPK-MM, 5 to 70 units/liter.

Abnormal results
Detectable CPK-BB levels may indicate brain tissue injury, certain widespread malignant tumors, severe shock, or renal failure. However, such elevations don't confirm a specific diagnosis.

CPK-MB levels above 5% of total CPK (or more than 10 units/liter) suggest an MI, especially if the lactate dehydrogenase isoenzyme ratio (LDH_1-LDH_2) exceeds 1. With an acute MI or cardiac surgery, CPK-MB levels begin rising in 2 to 4 hours, peak in 12 to 24 hours, and usually return to normal in 24 to 48 hours. Persistent elevations or increasing levels indicate ongoing myocardial damage. Total CPK levels follow roughly the same pattern but rise slightly later. Serious skeletal muscle injury that occurs in certain muscular dystrophies, polymyositis, and severe myoglobinuria may produce slightly elevated CPK-MB levels.

Rising CPK-MM values follow skeletal muscle damage from trauma, such as surgery and I.M. injection. Levels may be 50 to 100 times normal in such diseases as dermatomyositis and muscular dystrophy. Sharp elevations also occur with muscular activity caused by agitation, such as an acute psychotic episode. A moderate rise in CPK-MM levels develops in patients with hypothyroidism.

Elevated total CPK levels may occur in patients with severe hypokalemia, carbon monoxide poisoning, malignant hyperthermia, and alcoholic cardiomyopathy. Occasionally, total CPK levels rise following a pulmonary or cerebral infarction. CPK levels also increase after seizures.

Nursing implications of abnormal results

Your actions will vary according to the test results.

Increased CPK-MB levels. Assess the patient for signs and symptoms of an acute MI, including chest pain, dyspnea, cold and clammy skin, pallor, anxiety, and arrhythmias. Encourage the patient to rest, and alleviate chest discomfort with medications, as ordered.

Compare CPK-MB levels with levels of aspartate aminotransferase (AST) and LDH, enzymes whose levels also increase after myocardial damage. Periodically check serum levels of CPK-MB. If they suddenly increase again after leveling off, tell the doctor. This may signal an ex-

tension of the infarction.

Increased CPK-MM levels. Prepare the patient for a battery of tests to discover the specific muscle disease causing the muscle damage.

Creatinine, serum

A quantitative analysis of serum creatinine levels, this test provides a more sensitive measure of renal damage than blood urea nitrogen (BUN) levels do. That's because renal impairment is virtually the only cause of elevated serum creatinine levels.

Creatinine, a nonprotein end product of creatine metabolism, appears in serum in amounts proportional to the body's muscle mass. The kidneys easily excrete creatinine, with little or no tubular reabsorption. So creatinine levels are directly related to the glomerular filtration rate. Because creatinine levels normally remain constant, elevated levels usually indicate diminished renal function.

Purpose
● To assess renal glomerular filtration
● To screen for renal damage.

Procedure-related nursing care
Explain the test's purpose to the patient, and tell him you'll need a blood sample. Instruct him to restrict food and fluid intake for about 8 hours before the test.

Perform a venipuncture, using a 10- to 15-ml red-top tube.

Reference values
Serum creatinine levels in men range from 0.8 to 1.2 mg/dl (71 to

106 μmol/L); in women, from 0.6 to 0.9 mg/dl (53 to 80 μmol/L).

Abnormal results
Elevated serum creatinine levels generally indicate renal disease that has damaged at least 50% of the nephrons. Decreased levels may result from a loss of muscle mass in advanced muscular dystrophy.

Nursing implications of abnormal results
If the patient has an elevated serum creatinine level, check his BUN level. An increase in both suggests renal disease rather than an interfering substance in the test.

Assess his level of consciousness because confusion may accompany azotemia. If he becomes confused, take safety precautions. Also monitor fluid intake and output. Report a urine output of less than 30 ml/hour. Teach the patient to follow a protein-restricted diet, if ordered.

Creatinine clearance

An excellent diagnostic indicator of renal function, the creatinine clearance test determines how efficiently the kidneys clear creatinine from the blood. The rate of clearance is expressed in terms of the volume of blood (in milliliters) that the kidneys can clear of creatinine in 1 minute. The test requires a blood sample and a timed urine specimen.

Creatinine, the chief metabolite of creatine, is formed and excreted in constant amounts, with production proportional to total muscle mass. Normal physical activity, diet, and urine volume have little effect on this production, although strenuous exercise and a high-protein diet can

affect it. (For more information, see *Urine creatinine test.*)

Purpose
• To assess renal function (primarily glomerular filtration)
• To monitor the progression of renal insufficiency.

Procedure-related nursing care
Explain the test's purpose to the patient. Tell him that you'll need a timed urine specimen and at least one blood sample. Describe the urine collection procedure. Also, tell him to avoid eating an excessive amount of meat before the procedure and to avoid strenuous exercise during the urine collection period.

Collect a timed urine specimen for a 2-, 6-, 12-, or 24-hour period, as ordered. Anytime during this period, perform a venipuncture, collecting the blood sample in a 7-ml red-top tube.

Collect the urine specimen in a bottle containing a preservative to prevent creatinine degradation. Refrigerate the urine specimen or keep it on ice during the collection period. At the end of the period, send the specimen to the laboratory. Then tell the patient he may resume his normal diet and activities.

Reference values
For men at age 20, the creatinine clearance rate should be 90 ml/minute/1.73 m^2 of body surface. For women at age 20, the creatinine clearance rate should be 84 ml/minute/1.73 m^2. Clearance declines by 6 ml/minute/decade.

Abnormal results
A low creatinine clearance rate may result from reduced renal blood flow (from shock or renal artery obstruction), acute tubular necrosis, acute

or chronic glomerulonephritis, advanced bilateral renal lesions (as in polycystic kidney disease, renal tuberculosis, or cancer), or nephrosclerosis. Congestive heart failure and severe dehydration may also cause the creatinine clearance rate to drop.

An elevated creatinine clearance rate usually has little diagnostic significance.

Nursing implications of abnormal results

Assess the patient with a decreased creatinine clearance rate for signs and symptoms of deteriorating renal function, including reduced urine output and an altered level of consciousness from accumulating uremic toxins.

Erythrocyte sedimentation rate

A sensitive but nonspecific test, the erythrocyte sedimentation rate (ESR) commonly provides the earliest indication of disease when other chemical or physical signs are still normal. The rate typically rises significantly in widespread inflammatory disorders caused by infection or autoimmune mechanisms. Localized inflammation and cancer may prolong the ESR elevation.

The test measures the time needed for erythrocytes (red blood cells) in a whole blood sample to settle to the bottom of a vertical tube. As the erythrocytes descend in the tube, they displace an equal volume of plasma upward, which retards the downward progress of other settling blood elements. Factors affecting the ESR include the

Urine creatinine test

Though less precise than the creatinine clearance test, the urine creatinine test may be ordered to help assess glomerular filtration.

Procedure-related nursing care
As with the creatinine clearance test, advise the patient to avoid eating an excessive amount of meat before the test and to refrain from strenuous physical exercise during the collection period. Collect a 24-hour urine specimen in a bottle containing a preservative to prevent creatinine degradation. Refrigerate the specimen or keep it on ice during the collection period.

Reference values
Urine creatinine levels normally range from 1 to 1.9 g/day (7 to 14 mmol/d) for men and from 0.8 to 1.7 g/day (6 to 13 mmol/d) for women.

Abnormal results
Diminished levels may result from impaired renal perfusion (associated with shock, for example), renal disease (such as chronic glomerulonephritis), or urinary tract infection (as occurs in benign prostatic hyperplasia). Urine levels may also drop along with serum levels in disorders that decrease muscle mass, such as muscular dystrophy.

Increased levels usually have little diagnostic significance.

volume, surface area, density, aggregation, and surface charge of the erythrocytes. Plasma proteins (notably fibrinogen and globulin) promote aggregation, increasing the ESR.

Purpose
● To aid in diagnosing occult disease, such as tuberculosis, tissue necrosis, and connective tissue disease

• To monitor inflammatory and malignant disease.

Procedure-related nursing care

Explain the test's purpose to the patient, and tell him you'll need a blood sample. Perform a venipuncture, collecting the sample in a 7-ml lavender-top, 4.5-ml black-top, or 4.5-ml blue-top tube, depending on laboratory preference.

Examine the sample for clots and clumps, then send it to the laboratory immediately. The sample must be tested within 2 hours because the sedimentation rate decreases over time.

Reference values

The ESR ranges from 0 to 20 mm/hour; it increases with age.

Abnormal results

The ESR rises in most anemias, pregnancy, acute or chronic inflammation, tuberculosis, paraproteinemias (especially multiple myeloma and Waldenström's macroglobulinemia), rheumatic fever, rheumatoid arthritis, and some types of cancer.

Polycythemia, sickle cell anemia, hyperviscosity, and low plasma protein levels tend to depress the ESR.

Nursing implications of abnormal results

If an undiagnosed patient has an increased ESR, anticipate further tests to determine the cause, and prepare the patient as ordered.

An increased ESR in a patient being monitored for a change in an inflammatory process — rheumatoid arthritis, for instance — may signal the need for further treatment, such as medication and bed rest. A decreased ESR in such a patient means the inflammation has diminished. Reevaluate his care plan to allow for more activity.

Glucose, fasting plasma

Also known as the fasting blood sugar test, the fasting plasma glucose test is commonly used to screen for glucose metabolism disorders — primarily diabetes mellitus. This test measures the patient's plasma glucose levels after an 8- to 12-hour fast.

When a patient fasts, his plasma glucose levels decrease, stimulating the release of the hormone glucagon. This hormone raises plasma glucose levels by accelerating glycogenolysis, stimulating gluconeogenesis, and inhibiting glycogen synthesis. Normally, the secretion of insulin stops the rise in glucose levels. In patients with diabetes, however, the absence or deficiency of insulin allows persistently elevated glucose levels.

Purpose

• To screen for diabetes mellitus and other glucose metabolism disorders
• To monitor drug or dietary therapy in patients with diabetes mellitus
• To help determine the insulin requirements of patients who have uncontrolled diabetes mellitus and those who require parenteral or enteral nutritional support
• To help evaluate patients with known or suspected hypoglycemia.

Procedure-related nursing care

Explain the purpose of the test to the patient. Tell him it requires a blood sample and that he must fast, taking only water for 8 to 12 hours before the test.

If the patient is known to have diabetes, you should draw his blood before he receives insulin or an oral antidiabetic drug. Tell him to watch for symptoms of hypoglycemia, such as weakness, restlessness, nervousness, hunger, and sweating. Stress that he should report such symptoms immediately.

Prepare the laboratory slip for the blood sample with the time of the patient's last pretest meal and pretest medication, such as insulin or an oral antidiabetic drug. Also record the time the sample is collected.

Perform a venipuncture, collecting the sample in a 5-ml gray-top tube. If the sample can't be sent to the laboratory immediately, refrigerate it and transport it as soon as possible.

Give the patient a balanced meal or snack after the procedure. Assure him that he can now eat and take medications withheld before the procedure.

Reference values

The normal range for fasting plasma glucose levels will vary according to the procedure. Generally, after an 8- to 12-hour fast, normal values are between 70 and 115 mg/dl (3.89 to 6.11 mmol/L).

Abnormal results

Fasting plasma glucose levels greater than 115 mg/dl, but less than 140 mg/dl (7.7 mmol/L), may suggest impaired glucose tolerance. Levels greater than or equal to 140 mg/dl (obtained on two or more occasions) may indicate diabetes mellitus — if other causes of the patient's hyperglycemia have been ruled out.

Elevated levels can also result from pancreatitis, recent acute illness (such as myocardial infarction), Cushing's syndrome, pituitary adenoma, pancreatitis, hyperthyroidism, and pheochromocytoma. Hyperglycemia may also stem from

chronic hepatic disease, brain trauma, chronic illness, or chronic malnutrition and is typical in eclampsia, anoxia, and seizure disorders.

Depressed plasma glucose levels can result from hyperinsulinism (overdose of insulin being the most common cause), insulinoma, von Gierke's disease, functional or reactive hypoglycemia, hypothyroidism, adrenocortical insufficiency, congenital adrenal hyperplasia, hypopituitarism, islet cell carcinoma of the pancreas, hepatic necrosis, and glycogen storage disease.

Nursing implications of abnormal results

If the test reveals high glucose levels, observe the patient for signs and symptoms of hyperglycemia, including weight loss and excessive thirst, hunger, and urination.

If the patient's levels are low, you should observe for signs and symptoms of hypoglycemia, including confusion, weakness, and tachycardia.

If diabetes mellitus is suspected, but test results are borderline, anticipate additional glucose testing procedures.

Glucose tolerance test, oral

The most sensitive method of evaluating borderline diabetes mellitus, the oral glucose tolerance test measures carbohydrate metabolism after ingestion of a challenge dose of glucose. This test may not be used for patients with fasting plasma glucose values greater than 140 mg/dl (7.7 mmol/L) or postprandial plasma glucose values greater than 200 mg/dl (11.1 mmol/L).

With this test, the body rapidly absorbs the glucose, causing plasma glucose levels to rise and peak 30 minutes to 1 hour after ingestion. The pancreas responds by secreting more insulin, causing glucose levels to return to normal within 2 hours. During this period, plasma glucose levels are monitored to assess insulin secretion and the body's ability to metabolize glucose. Occasionally, levels are monitored for an additional 2 to 3 hours to aid diagnosis of hypoglycemia and malabsorption syndrome.

If the oral glucose tolerance test is performed on a patient with non-insulin-dependent diabetes (Type II), his fasting plasma glucose levels may be within the normal range. However, insufficient secretion of insulin after ingestion of carbohydrates will cause his plasma glucose levels to rise sharply and return to normal slowly. This decreased tolerance for glucose helps confirm non-insulin-dependent diabetes.

The oral glucose tolerance test shouldn't be performed on a person who's suspected of having insulinoma because prolonged fasting by such a patient can lead to fainting and coma.

Purpose
• To confirm diabetes mellitus in selected patients
• To aid in diagnosing hypoglycemia and malabsorption syndrome.

Procedure-related nursing care
Take the following actions before, during, and after the procedure.

Before the procedure. Explain the purpose of the test to the patient, and tell him that it requires several blood samples and a urine specimen.

Instruct him to maintain a high-carbohydrate diet, not to smoke, and to avoid caffeine and alcohol for 3 days before the test. Tell him to fast for 10 to 16 hours before the test and to avoid strenuous exercise for 8 hours before and during the test. Suggest that he bring a book or other quiet diversion with him because the procedure usually takes several hours.

Alert the patient to the symptoms of hypoglycemia — weakness, restlessness, nervousness, hunger, and sweating — and tell him to report such symptoms immediately.

Prepare the laboratory slip, specifying the time of the patient's last meal and the times of the blood sample collections. Also note the time of the patient's last pretest insulin or oral antidiabetic dose, if appropriate.

During the procedure. Obtain a fasting blood sample by performing a venipuncture — usually between 7 and 9 a.m. Draw the sample into a 7-ml gray-top tube. Collect a urine specimen at the same time, if appropriate.

After collecting these samples, administer the test load of oral glucose. Record the time when the patient starts drinking the solution. Encourage him to drink it all within 5 minutes.

You'll need to draw blood samples 30 minutes, 1 hour, 1½ hours, 2 hours, and 3 hours after the loading dose, as ordered. Use 7-ml gray-top tubes.

Tell the patient to lie down if he feels faint. If he develops severe hypoglycemia, draw a blood sample, record the time on the laboratory slip, and discontinue the test. Administer I.V. glucose or have the patient drink a glass of orange juice to reverse the reaction.

Interpreting abnormal plasma glucose results

The lists below give you the diagnostic criteria for diabetes mellitus, impaired glucose tolerance, and gestational diabetes.

Diabetes mellitus

In *nonpregnant adults*, diagnosis is restricted to those who have one of the following:
☐ random plasma glucose level ≥200 mg/dl plus classic signs and symptoms of diabetes mellitus, including polydipsia, polyuria, ketonuria, polyphagia, and rapid weight loss
☐ fasting plasma glucose level ≥140 mg/dl on at least two occasions
☐ fasting plasma glucose level <140 mg/dl, plus sustained elevated plasma glucose levels on at least two oral glucose tolerance test samples drawn within 2 hours.

In *chiidren*, diagnosis is restricted to those who have one of the following:
☐ random plasma glucose level ≥200 mg/dl plus classic signs and symptoms of diabetes mellitus, including polydipsia, polyuria, ketonuria, polyphagia, and rapid weight loss
☐ fasting plasma glucose level ≥140 mg/dl on at least two occasions and sustained elevated plasma glucose levels on at least two oral glucose tolerance test samples. Both the 2-hour plasma glucose levels and at least one other plasma sample taken between 0 and 2 hours after a patient receives the glucose dose (1.75 g/kg of ideal body weight up to 75 g) should be ≥200 mg/dl.

Impaired glucose tolerance

In *nonpregnant adults*, diagnosis is restricted to those who have all of the following:
☐ fasting plasma glucose level >115 mg/dl but <140 mg/dl
☐ 2-hour oral glucose tolerance test that yields a plasma glucose level between 140 and 200 mg/dl
☐ intervening oral glucose tolerance test that yields a plasma glucose level ≥200 mg/dl.

In *children*, diagnosis is restricted to those who have both of the following:
☐ fasting plasma glucose concentration >115 mg/dl but <140 mg/dl
☐ 2-hour oral glucose tolerance test that yields a plasma glucose level >140 mg/dl.

Gestational diabetes

In *pregnant women*, after an oral glucose load of 100 g, diagnosis may be made if two plasma glucose values equal or exceed:
☐ fasting value of 105 mg/dl
☐ 1-hour value of 190 mg/dl
☐ 2-hour value of 165 mg/dl
☐ 3-hour value of 145 mg/dl.

Send all blood and urine samples to the laboratory immediately. If you can't arrange to get the samples there immediately, refrigerate them and transport them as soon as possible.

After the procedure. Provide a balanced meal or a snack, observing the patient for signs and symptoms of a hypoglycemic reaction. Tell the patient to resume the diet and activities that were discontinued before the test.

Reference values

Normally, plasma glucose levels peak at 160 to 180 mg/dl (8.9 to 10 mmol/L) 30 minutes to 1 hour after administration of an oral glucose test dose and return to fasting levels (or lower) within 2 hours. Normal levels are less than 140 mg/dl (7.7 mmol/L) after 2 hours.

Abnormal results

If the 2-hour sample and at least one other sample (taken between 0 and 2 hours after a 75-g or greater glucose dose) show a glucose level greater than or equal to 200 mg/dl (11.1 mmol/L), this test confirms diabetes in a nonpregnant adult. (See *Interpreting abnormal plasma glucose results,* page 39.)

Increased glucose levels are associated with other serious conditions, such as Cushing's syndrome, pheochromocytoma, central nervous system lesions, cirrhosis of the liver, myocardial or cerebral infarction, hyperthyroidism, and anxiety states, as well as pregnancy.

Decreased glucose levels occur in hyperinsulinism, malabsorption syndrome, adrenocortical insufficiency (Addison's disease), hypothyroidism, and hypopituitarism.

Nursing implications of abnormal results

If the oral glucose tolerance test confirms a diagnosis of diabetes mellitus, initiate a comprehensive patient-teaching program, including diet, medications, exercise, and prevention of complications.

If the glucose level is below normal, and hyperinsulinism is suspected or confirmed, monitor the patient for hypoglycemia.

Glucose, 2-hour postprandial plasma

A screening test for diabetes mellitus, the 2-hour postprandial plasma glucose test requires a blood sample drawn 2 hours after the patient eats a meal. The results reflect the metabolic response to a carbohydrate challenge. Normally, the blood glucose level will return to the fasting level within 2 hours.

Purpose

- To monitor drug or diet therapy in patients with diabetes mellitus
- To identify disorders associated with abnormal glucose metabolism
- To confirm diabetes mellitus in patients with the classic signs and symptoms of the disorder.

Procedure-related nursing care

Explain the purpose of the test to the patient. Tell him it requires a blood sample drawn 2 hours after a meal. Instruct him to fast overnight (except for water) and then to eat a high-carbohydrate breakfast that includes milk, orange juice, cereal with sugar, and toast. Stress that he should avoid smoking and strenuous exercise after the meal.

Prepare the laboratory slip with the time of the patient's meal, the sample collection time, and the time the last pretest insulin or antidiabetic dose was given, if appropriate.

Perform a venipuncture, collecting the sample in a 5-ml gray-top tube. If you can't send the sample to the laboratory immediately, place it in the refrigerator and transport it as soon as possible.

Tell the patient he may resume eating and other activities that were discontinued before the test.

Reference values

Normal glucose values are less than or equal to 120 mg/dl (6.7 mmol/L) up to age 30. After that, the speed of glucose tolerance declines and levels may increase an average of 6 mg/dl for each decade over age 30.

Abnormal results

Values greater than 140 mg/dl are abnormal in adults under age 50; values greater than 160 mg/dl are abnormal in adults over age 60. A value greater than or equal to 200 mg/dl, plus the presence of the classic signs and symptoms of diabetes mellitus, confirms a diagnosis of diabetes mellitus.

Other causes of elevated glucose levels include the following conditions: pancreatitis, Cushing's syndrome, acromegaly, pheochromocytoma, chronic hepatic disease, nephrotic syndrome, gastrectomy with dumping syndrome, and seizure disorders.

Depressed glucose levels occur in hyperinsulinism, insulinoma, von Gierke's disease, functional or reactive hypoglycemia, hypothyroidism, adrenocortical insufficiency, congenital adrenal hyperplasia, hypopituitarism, islet cell carcinoma of the pancreas, hepatic necrosis, and glycogen storage disease.

Nursing implications of abnormal results

If the 2-hour postprandial plasma glucose test confirms a diagnosis of diabetes mellitus, initiate a comprehensive patient-teaching program, including diet, medications, exercise, and prevention of complications.

Glycosylated hemoglobin

A diagnostic tool for monitoring diabetes therapy, the glycosylated hemoglobin test measures three minor hemoglobins (Hb): A_{1a}, A_{1b}, and A_{1c}. These three hemoglobins are variants of Hb A formed by glycosylation—a nearly irreversible molecular process in which glucose becomes chemically incorporated in Hb A. Because glycosylation occurs at a constant rate during the 120-day life span of a red blood cell (RBC), glycosylated hemoglobin levels reflect the average blood glucose level during the preceding 6 to 10 weeks. This makes the test most appropriate for evaluating the long-term effectiveness of a patient's diabetes therapy.

The glycosylated hemoglobin test has distinct advantages over the traditional blood or urine glucose tests. For example, the blood test requires repeated venipunctures, and each measurement reflects the patient's glucose control only at the moment the sample was taken. The urine test also reflects the patient's glucose control only at the time of collection. In contrast, the glycosylated hemoglobin test requires only one venipuncture every 6 to 8 weeks and accurately reflects diabetes control over the preceding 6 to 10 weeks.

Purpose

• To monitor control of diabetes mellitus.

Procedure-related nursing care

Explain the purpose of the test to the patient, and tell him it requires a blood sample. Instruct him to maintain his prescribed medication or diet regimen before the procedure.

Perform a venipuncture, collecting the sample in a 5-ml lavender-top tube. Be sure that you completely fill the collection tube. Then invert it gently several times so that you mix the sample and the anticoagulant adequately.

After the test, schedule the patient for appropriate follow-up testing in 6 to 8 weeks.

Reference values

Glycosylated hemoglobin values are reported as a percentage of the total hemoglobin within an RBC. Because Hb A_{1c} is present in a larger quantity than the other minor hemoglobins, it's the variant commonly measured. Reference values for Hb A_{1c} are usually 6% to 8% of the total hemoglobin within an RBC.

Abnormal results

If Hb A_{1c} accounts for more than 8% of the total hemoglobin within an RBC, the patient's diabetes mellitus isn't considered under control.

Nursing implications of abnormal results

If the glycosylated hemoglobin results are elevated, assess the patient's compliance with his diabetes mellitus treatment plan. If necessary, reinforce patient teaching or provide counseling. If the patient is complying with his treatment program, he may need adjustments in his diet or medication. Provide patient teaching according to new medical orders.

Hematocrit

A common test, hematocrit (HCT) measures the percentage of packed red blood cells (RBCs) in a whole blood sample. Thus, an HCT of 40% (0.40) means that a 100-ml sample contains 40 ml of packed RBCs. HCT depends mainly on the number of RBCs but is also influenced by the size of the average RBC. Therefore, conditions that result in elevated concentrations of blood glucose and sodium (which cause swelling of RBCs) may produce elevated HCT. This test may be automatically performed as part of the complete blood count (CBC). (See *What the CBC reveals*.)

What the CBC reveals

A common test, the complete blood count (CBC) provides a fairly complete picture of all the blood's formed elements.

What's tested

Typically, the CBC includes these components: hemoglobin concentration, hematocrit, red blood cell (RBC) and white blood cell (WBC) counts, WBC differential, and stained RBC examination.

What the results indicate

Besides pointing the way toward further definitive studies, the CBC also provides valuable information to help detect anemias and determine their severity, and to compare the status of specific blood elements. This makes the CBC especially useful for evaluating conditions in which the hematocrit doesn't parallel the RBC count, such as microcytic or macrocytic anemia.

Also part of the CBC, the stained RBC examination is commonly done with the WBC differential. After the differential, the same stained slide is evaluated for RBC distribution and morphology—including changes in cell contents, color, size, and shape. This provides more information for detecting leukemia, anemia, and thalassemia. Variations in the size and shape of RBCs are reported as occasional, slight, moderate, marked, or very marked; structural variations are reported as the number of immature or nucleated RBCs per 100 WBCs. Cell inclusions are also noted.

Purpose
- To aid diagnosis of abnormal states of hydration, polycythemia, and anemia
- To aid in calculating RBC indices
- To monitor fluid imbalance
- To monitor blood loss and evaluate blood replacement.

Procedure-related nursing care
Explain the purpose of the test to the patient, and tell him it requires a blood sample drawn from his finger. The blood sample may be drawn from the earlobe of a child, or the great toe or heel of an infant or a child.

Perform a fingerstick on an adult, using a heparinized capillary tube with a red band on the anticoagulant end. Fill the capillary tube from the red-banded end to about two-thirds capacity, and seal this end with clay.

Reference values
HCT values vary, depending on the patient's sex and age, the type of sample, and the laboratory performing the test. Reference values range from 40% to 54% (0.40 to 0.54) for men and from 37% to 47% (0.37 to 0.47) for women.

Abnormal results
High HCT suggests polycythemia or hemoconcentration caused by blood loss; low HCT may indicate anemia or hemodilution.

Nursing implications of abnormal results
When a patient has increased HCT, assess him for signs and symptoms of dehydration, such as thirst, decreased urine output, and poor skin turgor. Administer I.V. or oral fluids, as ordered.

Assess a patient with decreased HCT for signs and symptoms of ane-mia, such as pallor, tachycardia, and fatigue. If significant blood loss is also suspected, assess for signs and symptoms of shock, such as tachycardia, hypotension, rapid respirations, and cold, clammy skin.

Hemoglobin, total

Usually done as part of the complete blood count, this test measures the

Urine hemoglobin test

Aging red blood cells (RBCs) are constantly being destroyed by normal mechanisms within the reticuloendothelial system. But when RBC destruction occurs within the circulation—as in intravascular hemolysis—free hemoglobin (Hb) enters the plasma and binds with haptoglobin, a plasma alpha$_2$ globulin. If the plasma level of Hb exceeds that of haptoglobin, the excess unbound Hb is excreted in the urine.

Procedure-related nursing care
Inform the patient that the test requires a random urine specimen. Teach him the proper collection technique.

If a female patient is menstruating, reschedule the test because contamination of the specimen with menstrual blood alters test results.

Normal results
Normally, Hb doesn't appear in urine.

Abnormal results
Hemoglobinuria may occur in hemolytic anemias; in severe intravascular hemolysis, such as from a transfusion reaction; or when renal epithelial damage exists, such as in acute glomerulonephritis.

Hemoglobin reference values

AGE GROUP	REFERENCE VALUE
Less than 1 week old	17 to 22 g/dl
1 week old	15 to 20 g/dl
1 month old	11 to 15 g/dl
Child (5 to 14 years)	11 to 13 g/dl
Adult male	14 to 18 g/dl
Adult female	12 to 16 g/dl

grams of hemoglobin (Hb) found in a deciliter (100 ml) of whole blood. Hb concentration correlates closely with the red blood cell (RBC) count and is affected by the Hb-RBC ratio and free plasma hemoglobin levels. (Also see *Urine hemoglobin test,* page 43.)

Purpose
• To measure the severity of anemia or polycythemia
• To monitor the patient's response to therapy for anemia.

Procedure-related nursing care
Explain the test's purpose to the patient, and tell him it requires a blood sample. As appropriate, explain to the patient's parents that a small amount of blood will be drawn from the finger or earlobe of a child, or the great toe or heel of an infant.

Perform a venipuncture on an adult or older child, collecting the sample in a 7-ml lavender-top tube. For an infant or a young child, collect capillary blood in a pipette.

Reference values
Normal Hb concentrations vary according to the patient's age and sex and the type of blood sample drawn. Remember, the values for infants and children are based on a capillary sample; values for all other patients are based on a venous blood sample (see *Hemoglobin reference values*).

Abnormal results
An elevated Hb level suggests hemoconcentration from polycythemia or dehydration. A low concentration of Hb may indicate anemia, recent hemorrhage, or fluid retention, causing hemodilution.

Nursing implications of abnormal results
If the Hb level is elevated, observe the patient for signs and symptoms of dehydration, such as marked thirst, poor skin turgor, dry mucous membranes, and shocklike symptoms. Ensure that the patient receives adequate fluid.

With decreased Hb levels, observe the patient for signs and symptoms of anemia, such as dizziness, tachycardia, weakness, and dyspnea at rest. Also check the patient's hematocrit because it, too, may be low.

If diet is considered a cause of decreased Hb, provide instructions for a diet that stresses increased iron intake.

Hepatitis B surface antigen

The earliest and most reliable serologic marker of viral hepatitis infection, the hepatitis B surface antigen (HBsAg) appears in the serum of a patient with hepatitis B virus (HBV) as early as 14 days after exposure and throughout an acute illness.

HBsAg can be detected by radio-immunoassay. Less commonly, it's detected by reverse passive hemagglutination during the extended incubation period and through the first 3 weeks of acute infection. The antigen can also be detected in a carrier's blood.

After donation, all blood is screened for HBV before it's stored. This screening, required by the Food and Drug Administration, has reduced the incidence of hepatitis. However, the test doesn't screen for hepatitis A or C (non-A, non-B) viruses.

Purpose
- To screen blood for HBV
- To screen persons at high risk for contracting HBV, such as hemodialysis nurses
- To aid differential diagnosis of viral hepatitis.

Procedure-related nursing care
Explain the purpose of the test to the patient, and tell him that it requires a blood sample.

Perform the venipuncture, using a 7-ml red-top tube to collect the sample. Because this is a blood-borne infection, take extra care, following blood and body fluid precautions. Make sure you:
- wear gloves
- avoid accidental needle puncture
- wash your hands after the procedure
- dispose of the needle properly.

If you accidentally stick yourself with a used needle, report the incident immediately. Expect to receive gamma globulin to help prevent the disease.

Normal results
Serum is normally negative for HBsAg.

Abnormal results
The presence of HBsAg in a patient with hepatitis confirms hepatitis B. In chronic carriers and persons with chronic active hepatitis, HBsAg may be present in serum several months after the onset of acute infection. HBsAg may also occur in more than 5% of patients with certain diseases other than hepatitis, such as hemophilia, Hodgkin's disease, and leukemia.

Nursing implications of abnormal results
Notify the blood donor if he tests positive for HBsAg. In most states, you need to report cases of confirmed viral hepatitis to public health authorities.

Also, assess the patient for signs and symptoms of hepatitis, such as jaundice, anorexia, fever, dark-colored urine, pain in the right upper abdominal quadrant, and nausea and vomiting. If you note these signs, report them immediately to the doctor. Encourage the patient to get plenty of rest, to eat nutritious meals, and to drink plenty of fluids—especially fruit juices.

If the test confirms a diagnosis of hepatitis, follow your hospital's isolation procedure.

HIV antibody: Serum enzyme immunoassay

This enzyme immunoassay detects the presence of the antibody to human immunodeficiency virus (HIV) antigen. This antibody develops in response to HIV exposure, usually within 6 to 8 weeks. Occasionally, a longer period exists between exposure and development of the anti-

What happens in HIV replication

In acquired immunodeficiency syndrome (AIDS), the number of CD4 T cells declines, mainly because the human immunodeficiency virus (HIV) selectively binds with and destroys them. This destructive process begins as a protein on the viral envelope, called gp 120, binds tightly with the CD4 receptor, a protein found on the CD4 T cell's surface. The virus then fuses with the cell membrane and enters the cell. Once inside, the virus sheds its inner protein coat. Then, with the help of the enzyme reverse transcriptase, it copies the genetic instructions of a strand of HIV RNA as a double-stranded DNA. This DNA then enters the nucleus of the CD4 T cell, where it's incorporated into the genetic material. At this point, HIV's replication cycle may be suspended until the CD4 T cell becomes activated.

Activating the CD4 T cell

CD4 T cells can be activated by such pathogens as cytomegalovirus, Epstein-Barr virus, hepatitis A and B viruses, and herpes simplex virus. They can also be stimulated allogeneically by exposure to such body fluids as semen or blood. Once activation occurs, transcription begins. In this process, an enzyme in the CD4 T cell copies the virus's DNA. These copies, called messenger HIV RNA, leave the nucleus, carrying instructions for making new HIV. Protein synthesis—a process that produces the components of the new virus—follows. These components are then assembled into the new HIV, which buds from the CD4 T cell and breaks free as a mature HIV. This process kills the CD4 T cell.

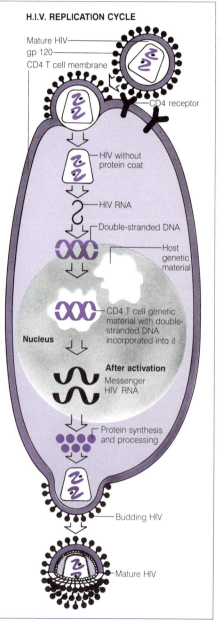

H.I.V. REPLICATION CYCLE

Mature HIV
gp 120
CD4 T cell membrane
CD4 receptor
HIV without protein coat
HIV RNA
Double-stranded DNA
Host genetic material
CD4 T cell genetic material with double-stranded DNA incorporated into it
Nucleus
After activation
Messenger HIV RNA
Protein synthesis and processing
Budding HIV
Mature HIV

body. Because this test is highly sensitive and specific, it's used routinely to screen for HIV infection and to test all donated blood. (See *What happens in HIV replication.*)

Purpose
- To aid diagnosis of HIV infection
- To detect exposure to HIV.

Procedure-related nursing care
Explain the purpose of the test to the patient, and tell him it requires a blood sample.

Perform the venipuncture, collecting the sample in a 7-ml red-top tube. Because HIV is a blood-borne infection, take extra care, following blood and body fluid precautions. Make sure you:
- wear gloves
- avoid accidental needle puncture
- wash your hands after the procedure
- dispose of the needle properly.

If you accidentally stick yourself with a used needle, report the incident immediately.

Normal results
Patients without the antibody will usually test negative.

Abnormal results
A positive test indicates exposure to HIV; it doesn't indicate that the patient currently has acquired immunodeficiency syndrome (AIDS). However, the patient will almost certainly develop AIDS within 10 years of exposure to the virus.

Occasionally, false-positive test results may occur in patients with autoimmune diseases, such as systemic lupus erythematosus, or in patients with antibodies to human leukocyte antigens. Also, in populations with a very low prevalence of HIV infection, a high percentage of false-positive test results may occur.

Nursing implications of abnormal results
Because false-positive results are possible, this immunoassay requires confirmation by another diagnostic test—such as the Western blot assay—before you can advise the patient on making major decisions regarding his life-style, health care, or precautions.

If the Western blot assay confirms the results of the immunoassay, counsel the patient and his sexual partner about preventing the spread of the virus. Advise him that any previous sexual partners or anyone who has shared a needle with him should also undergo testing and counseling.

HIV antibody: Western blot assay

This immunoblotting test detects antibodies to human immunodeficiency virus (HIV) particles by separating the HIV antigens according to their molecular weights. Once the antigens are separated, antibodies can be identified as reacting with specific antigens of particular molecular weights, known as bands. The appearance of specific bands confirms exposure to the HIV virus.

Purpose
- To confirm the presence of HIV antibodies in patients who have a positive enzyme immunoassay for HIV antibodies.

Procedure-related nursing care
Explain the purpose of the test, and tell the patient that it requires a blood sample.

Perform a venipuncture and col-

lect the sample in a 7-ml red-top tube. Because HIV is a blood-borne infection, follow blood and body fluid precautions. Make sure you:
- wear gloves
- avoid accidental needle puncture
- wash your hands after the procedure
- dispose of the needle properly.

If you accidentally stick yourself with a needle, report the incident immediately.

Normal results
Normally, the test is negative for HIV antibodies.

Abnormal results
A positive test confirms that the patient has antibodies to HIV. As with the enzyme immunoassay, a positive test result doesn't mean the patient has acquired immunodeficiency syndrome (AIDS), but he'll almost certainly develop it within 10 years of exposure to the virus. The duration between HIV exposure and the development of AIDS varies greatly.

Nursing implications of abnormal results
Tell the patient who tests positive that he should receive counseling and medical care to plan and carry out the most effective preventive therapy and treatment for AIDS and its complications. Explain that anyone who's had sexual contact or shared a needle with him should also be tested and counseled.

Human chorionic gonadotropin, urine

Commonly used to detect pregnancy, human chorionic gonadotropin (HCG) is a glycoprotein hormone produced by the trophoblastic cells of the placenta. Although its precise function is unclear, apparently HCG, along with progesterone, maintains the corpus luteum during early pregnancy.

Production of HCG increases steadily during the first trimester, peaking around the 10th week of gestation. Levels then fall to less than 10% of first trimester peak levels. (See *The role of human chorionic gonadotropin.*)

The qualitative analysis of HCG in the urine can detect pregnancy as early as 10 days after a missed menstrual period. Quantitative measurements may be used to evaluate a suspected hydatidiform mole or HCG-secreting tumors.

Because it's easier to perform and less costly than the serum HCG test (beta-subunit assay), the qualitative urine HCG analysis is usually the test of choice to detect pregnancy. However, the serum HCG test can detect pregnancy as early as 7 days after conception (see *Serum HCG test*, page 50).

Purpose
- To detect and confirm pregnancy
- To aid the diagnosis of hydatidiform mole or HCG-secreting tumors.

Procedure-related nursing care
Explain the purpose of the test to the patient, and inform her that it requires a first-voided morning specimen for a qualitative analysis—or a 24-hour urine collection for a quantitative analysis.

Prepare the laboratory slip with the date of the patient's last menstrual period.

Collect the appropriate urine specimen. If you're collecting a 24-hour specimen, you must either refrigerate it or keep it on ice during

The role of human chorionic gonadotropin

Nine days after ovulation, the trophoblastic cells of the blastocyst begin secreting human chorionic gonadotropin (HCG) if implantation occurs. Under the influence of HCG, the corpus luteum secretes increasing amounts of estrogen and progesterone – vital for a successful pregnancy because these hormones promote early development of the endometrium, placenta, and fetus. The trophoblastic cells develop into the chorionic villi of the placenta and continue secreting HCG. Levels of HCG peak around the 10th week of gestation.

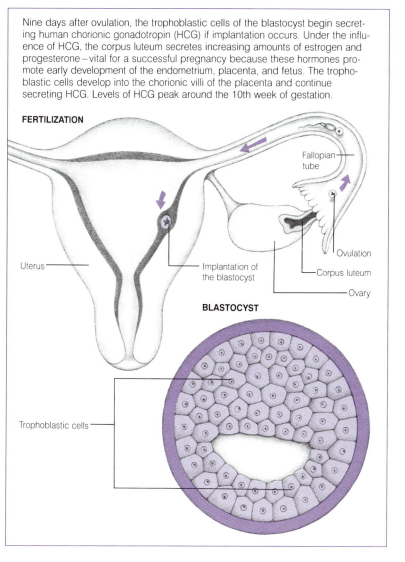

the entire collection period.

Normal results
In qualitative analysis, if agglutination fails to occur, test results are positive, indicating that the patient is pregnant.

In quantitative analysis, urine HCG levels in the first trimester of a normal pregnancy may be as high

Serum HCG test

This serum radioimmunoassay, a quantitative analysis of the HCG beta-subunit level, is much more sensitive and costly than the routine urine test ordered for pregnancy. However, it may be ordered:
• to detect early pregnancy or to determine the adequacy of hormone production in high-risk pregnancies
• to aid in diagnosing trophoblastic tumors, such as hydatidiform mole or choriocarcinoma, and tumors that secrete HCG ectopically
• to monitor treatment for induction of ovulation and conception.

Reference values
Values for serum HCG should be less than 3 IU/ml.

Abnormal results
Elevated serum HCG levels may indicate pregnancy; sharply elevated levels may indicate a multiple pregnancy. Increased levels may also indicate the presence of a tumor. However, the HCG beta-subunit levels can't differentiate between pregnancy and tumor recurrence.
   Low serum HCG beta-subunit levels can occur in ectopic pregnancy or pregnancy of less than 9 days.

as 500,000 IU/day; in the second trimester, they range from 10,000 to 25,000 IU/day; and in the third trimester, from 5,000 to 15,000 IU/day. After delivery, HCG levels decline rapidly, becoming undetectable within a few days.

You won't normally find measurable HCG in the urine of men or nonpregnant women.

Abnormal results
After the first trimester, elevated urine HCG levels may indicate multiple pregnancy or erythroblastosis fetalis. Depressed urine HCG levels may indicate threatened spontaneous abortion or ectopic pregnancy.

Measurable levels of HCG in men or nonpregnant women may indicate these conditions: choriocarcinoma, testicular or ovarian tumors, melanoma, multiple myeloma, or gastric, hepatic, pancreatic, or breast cancer.

Nursing implications of abnormal results
If the patient tests positive for pregnancy, advise her to seek appropriate medical care.

If a hydatidiform mole or HCG-secreting tumor is diagnosed, support the patient emotionally and reinforce the doctor's explanation as necessary. Prepare the patient for further ordered tests, such as Doppler ultrasonography and histologic studies.

Lactate dehydrogenase

An enzyme, lactate dehydrogenase (LDH) catalyzes the reversible conversion of muscle pyruvic acid into lactic acid. Because LDH appears in almost all body tissues, cellular damage causes an elevation of total serum LDH levels, thus limiting its diagnostic usefulness.

However, five tissue-specific isoenzymes can be identified and measured: LDH_1 and LDH_2 appear primarily in the heart, red blood cells, and kidneys; LDH_3, primarily in the lungs; and LDH_4 and LDH_5, in the liver and skeletal muscles. This test is widely used to detect myocardial infarction (MI) because the myocardial LDH level rises 12 to 48 hours after an MI begins, peaks in 2 to 5 days, and drops to normal in 7 to 14 days if tissue necrosis doesn't persist.

Purpose
• To aid differential diagnosis of MI, pulmonary infarction, anemias, and hepatic disease
• To support creatine phosphokinase (CPK) isoenzyme test results in diagnosing MI, or to help in diagnosing an MI when CPK-MB samples are drawn too late (more than 24 hours after the onset of acute MI)
• To monitor patient response to some forms of chemotherapy.

Procedure-related nursing care
Explain the purpose of the test to the patient, and tell him it requires a blood sample. If the patient is suspected of having experienced an MI, tell him that the test will be repeated on the next two mornings to monitor progressive changes.

Perform a venipuncture, collecting the sample in a 7-ml red-top tube. Draw each sample on schedule to avoid missing peak levels, and mark the collection time on the laboratory slip.

Send the sample to the laboratory immediately or, if transport is delayed, keep the sample at room temperature. Changes in temperature reportedly inactivate LDH_5, thus altering isoenzyme patterns.

Reference values
Total LDH levels should range from 48 to 115 units/liter. Distribution of isoenzymes should be as follows:
• LDH_1 — 17.5% to 28.3% of total
• LDH_2 — 30.4% to 36.4% of total
• LDH_3 — 19.2% to 24.8% of total
• LDH_4 — 9.6% to 15.6% of total
• LDH_5 — 5.5% to 12.7% of total.

Abnormal results
Because many common disorders raise total LDH levels, isoenzyme electrophoresis is usually required for diagnosis. (See *Interpreting LDH isoenzyme values.*)

Interpreting LDH isoenzyme values

This table shows the correlation between elevated isoenzyme levels (gray boxes) and probable diagnoses.

DISEASE	LDH_1	LDH_2	LDH_3	LDH_4	LDH_5
Cardiopulmonary					
Myocardial infarction	█	█			
Myocardial infarction with hepatic congestion	█	█			█
Rheumatic carditis	█	█			
Myocarditis	█	█			
Congestive heart failure (decompensated)				█	█
Shock	█			█	█
Pulmonary infarction			█		
Hematologic					
Pernicious anemia	█	█			
Hemolytic anemia	█	█			
Sickle cell anemia	█	█			
Gastrointestinal					
Hepatobiliary disorder					█
Hepatitis					█
Active cirrhosis					█
Hepatic congestion					█

In some disorders, total LDH may be within normal limits, but abnormal proportions of each isoenzyme indicate specific organ tissue damage. For instance, in acute MI the concentration of LDH_1 is greater than LDH_2 within 12 to 48 hours after the onset of symptoms. This reversal of the normal isoenzyme pattern typifies myocardial damage and is referred to as flipped LDH.

Nursing implications of abnormal results

When test results show a flipped LDH — and especially if the patient has a history of chest pain — a likely diagnosis is MI. Stress the importance of mental and physical rest, monitor cardiac status, and administer medications to relieve chest discomfort, as ordered.

Compare results with CPK and aspartate aminotransferase (AST) findings.

Lipoprotein-cholesterol fractionation

Cholesterol fractionation tests isolate and measure the cholesterol in serum — low-density lipoproteins (LDLs) and high-density lipoproteins (HDLs). Cholesterol in LDL and HDL fractions is considered significant since the Framingham Heart Study showed that the cholesterol level in HDL is inversely related to the incidence of coronary artery disease (CAD). Thus, the higher the HDL level, the lower the incidence of CAD. The higher the LDL level, the higher the incidence of CAD.

Purpose
• To assess the risk of CAD.

Procedure-related nursing care

Explain the purpose of the test to the patient, and tell him it requires a blood sample. Tell him to maintain his normal diet for 2 weeks before the test, to abstain from alcohol for 24 hours before the test, and to fast and avoid exercise for 12 to 14 hours before the test.

Perform a venipuncture, collecting the sample in a 7-ml red-top tube. Send the sample to the laboratory immediately; if that's not possible, place the sample in the refrigerator until you can transport it.

After the test, the patient may resume his diet and any activities restricted by the test.

Reference values

Normal HDL-cholesterol levels range from 29 to 77 mg/dl (0.8 to 2 mmol/L) and normal LDL-cholesterol levels range from 62 to 185 mg/dl (1.6 to 4.7 mmol/L). These values vary according to age, sex, geographic region, and ethnic group, so check with your laboratory for appropriate normal values.

Abnormal results

High LDL levels increase the risk of CAD. Elevated HDL levels generally reflect a healthy state but also can indicate chronic hepatitis, early-stage primary biliary cirrhosis, or alcohol consumption. Rarely, a sharp rise (one as high as 100 mg/dl) in a second type of HDL ($alpha_2$-HDL) may signal CAD.

Nursing implications of abnormal results

Teach the patient with an elevated LDL level to help reduce his risk of CAD by eating properly, controlling his weight, exercising, and avoiding smoking. Explain that exercise decreases LDL levels better than diet alone — and that the combination of a diet lower in LDL-cholesterol and increased activity is the best way to decrease LDL levels.

Magnesium, serum

This test, a quantitative analysis, measures serum levels of magnesium—the most abundant intracellular cation other than potassium. Vital to neuromuscular function, this often-overlooked electrolyte helps regulate intracellular metabolism, activates many essential enzymes, and affects the metabolism of nucleic acids and proteins. Magnesium also helps transport sodium and potassium across cell membranes and, through its effect on the secretion of parathyroid hormone, influences intracellular calcium levels.

Most magnesium is found in bone and in intracellular fluid; a small amount is found in extracellular fluid. Absorbed by the small intestine, magnesium is excreted in the urine and feces. (See *Urine magnesium test.*)

Purpose
• To evaluate electrolyte status
• To assess neuromuscular or renal function.

Procedure-related nursing care
Explain the purpose of the test to the patient, and tell him it requires a blood sample.

Perform a venipuncture, collecting the sample in a 10- to 15-ml red-top tube. About 75% of the blood's magnesium is in the red blood cells, so handle the sample gently to prevent hemolysis.

Reference values
Serum magnesium levels normally

Urine magnesium test

Measuring the urine level of magnesium over a 24-hour period has several advantages over the serum magnesium test. A relatively inexpensive and simple procedure, the urine test can detect a magnesium deficiency before serum magnesium levels change. As a result, the urine magnesium test is increasingly used to rule out magnesium deficiency as the cause of neurologic symptoms and to help evaluate glomerular function in suspected renal disease.

Reference values
Normal urinary excretion of magnesium is less than 150 mg/24 hours (6.2 mmol/d).

Abnormal results
Elevated urine magnesium levels may result from early chronic renal disease, adrenocortical insufficiency (Addison's disease), chronic alcoholism, or chronic ingestion of magnesium-containing antacids. Low urine magnesium levels may result from malabsorption, acute or chronic diarrhea, diabetic acidosis, dehydration, pancreatitis, advanced renal failure, primary aldosteronism, or decreased dietary intake of magnesium.

range from 1.8 to 2.4 mg/dl (0.7 to 1.2 mmol/L).

Abnormal results
Elevated serum magnesium levels (hypermagnesemia) most commonly occur in renal failure, when the kidneys excrete inadequate amounts of magnesium. Adrenocortical insufficiency (Addison's disease) can also elevate serum magnesium levels.

Decreased serum magnesium levels (hypomagnesemia) most commonly result from chronic alcoholism. Other causes include diarrhea, malabsorption syndrome, faulty absorption after bowel resection, prolonged bowel or gastric aspiration, acute pancreatitis, primary aldosteronism, severe burns, hypercalcemic conditions (including hyperparathyroidism), and certain diuretic therapies.

Nursing implications of abnormal results

If the patient shows increased magnesium levels, monitor him for signs of hypermagnesemia: lethargy; flushing; diaphoresis; decreased blood pressure; a slow, weak pulse rate; diminished deep tendon reflexes; muscle weakness; and slow, shallow respirations.

With decreased magnesium levels, watch the patient for signs of hypomagnesemia: leg and foot cramps, hyperactive deep tendon reflexes, cardiac arrhythmias, muscle weakness, seizures, twitching, tremors, and tetany.

Occult blood, fecal

Invisible because of its minute quantity, fecal occult blood can be

PROCEDURES

detected by microscopic analysis or by chemical tests for hemoglobin, such as the guaiac or orthotoluidine test. Normally, small amounts of blood (2 to 2.5 ml/day) appear in the feces. So these tests are designed to detect quantities greater than normal.

A fecal occult blood test is indicated in patients whose clinical symptoms and preliminary blood studies suggest GI bleeding. Further tests will pinpoint the exact origin of the bleeding. Particularly important for early diagnosis of colorectal cancer, the fecal occult blood test will be positive in 80% of persons with this cancer.

Purpose

• To detect GI bleeding
• To aid early diagnosis of colorectal cancer.

Procedure-related nursing care

Explain the purpose of the test to the patient. Tell him it requires three stool specimens. (Occasionally only one random specimen will be used.) Instruct him to avoid contaminating the stool specimen with toilet tissue or urine. Tell him to maintain a high-fiber diet and to avoid eating red meats, poultry,

Testing fecal specimens for occult blood

You can test a fecal specimen for occult blood by following these steps:
• Obtain small specimens from two different areas of each stool to allow for any variance in the distribution of blood.
• Place a specimen on a piece of filter paper.
• For the *guaiac test,* add two drops

each of tap water, glacial acid, 1:60 solution of gum guaiac in 95% ethyl alcohol, and 3% hydrogen peroxide.

For the *orthotoluidine test,* add two drops each of 0.2% orthotoluidine and 0.3% hydrogen peroxide.
• Mix thoroughly with a tongue blade. Note the color immediately, and check it again after 5 minutes.

fish, turnips, and horseradish for 48 to 72 hours before the test and throughout the collection period.

Collect three stool specimens or a random specimen, as appropriate. Send the specimen to the laboratory, or perform the test yourself, as ordered (see *Testing fecal specimens for occult blood*). The patient may resume his normal diet after the test.

Normal results
Normally, less than 2.5 ml of blood is present and the test will result in a green reaction.

Abnormal results
A dark blue reaction that appears within 5 minutes is a positive indication for fecal occult blood. If the blue appears within 3 to 4 minutes, consider it strongly positive; a faint blue reaction is weakly positive and not necessarily abnormal.

A positive test indicates GI bleeding that can result from several disorders, including varices, peptic ulcer, carcinoma, ulcerative colitis, dysentery, or hemorrhagic disease.

Nursing implications of abnormal results
If the sample is positive for occult blood, anticipate further tests, such as barium swallow, analyses of gastric contents, and endoscopic procedures to define the site and extent of bleeding.

Phosphates, serum

This test measures serum levels of phosphates, the dominant cellular anion. Phosphates help store and utilize body energy; they help regulate calcium levels, carbohydrate and lipid metabolism, and acid-base balance; and they're essential to bone formation (about 85% of the body's phosphates are found in bone).

The small intestine absorbs a considerable amount of phosphates from dietary sources, but adequate levels of vitamin D are necessary for the absorption of phosphates. The kidneys excrete phosphates and serve as a regulatory mechanism. Because calcium and phosphates interact in a reciprocal relationship, urinary excretion of phosphates increases or decreases in inverse proportion to serum calcium levels. Abnormal concentrations of phosphates result more often from improper excretion than they do from abnormal ingestion or absorption from dietary sources. (See *Urine phosphate test,* page 56.)

Purpose
• To aid the diagnosis of renal disorders and acid-base imbalance
• To detect endocrine, skeletal, and calcium disorders.

Procedure-related nursing care
Explain the purpose of the test to the patient, and tell him it requires a blood sample. Perform a venipuncture and collect the sample in a 10- to 15-ml red-top tube. Handle the sample gently to prevent hemolysis, which falsely increases phosphate levels.

Reference values
Serum phosphate levels normally range from 2.5 to 4.5 mg/dl (0.80 to 1.40 mmol/L) or from 1.8 to 2.6 mEq/liter. Children have higher serum phosphate levels than adults; their phosphate levels can rise as high as 7 mg/dl (2.25 mmol/L) during periods of increased bone growth.

Urine phosphate test

Generally, you can expect urine phosphate levels to parallel serum levels. This test, which requires a 24-hour urine specimen, is usually performed at the same time as a urine calcium test. The results are used to help evaluate phosphate metabolism and excretion and to monitor treatment of a phosphate deficiency. Factors that indirectly affect the urine phosphate level include parathyroid hormone, calcitonin, and plasma protein levels.

Procedure-related nursing care
Encourage the patient to be as active as possible before the test. Tell him to follow the Albright-Reefinstein diet (which contains about 130 mg of calcium/24 hours) for 3 days before the test. Have a dietitian explain this diet to him.

Reference values
Normal excretion of phosphates is < 1,000 mg/24 hours.

Abnormal results
Elevated urine phosphate levels are associated with hyperparathyroidism, renal tubular acidosis, and sometimes multiple myeloma. Decreased levels occur with vitamin D intoxication, sarcoidosis, hypoparathyroidism, chronic nephrosis, acute nephritis, osteomalacia, and steatorrhea.

Abnormal results
Because serum phosphate levels alone have limited diagnostic value (only a few rare conditions directly affect phosphate metabolism), they should be interpreted in light of serum calcium levels. Although rarely clinically significant, elevated phosphate levels may result from skeletal disease, healing fractures, hypoparathyroidism, acromegaly, diabetic acidosis, high intestinal obstruction, and renal failure. Depressed phosphate levels may result from malnutrition, malabsorption syndrome, hyperparathyroidism, renal tubular acidosis, or treatment of diabetic acidosis.

Nursing implications of abnormal results
If serum phosphate levels are increased, check the serum calcium level, which may be low. If so, observe for tetany. Monitor the patient's urine output; if it drops below 25 ml/hour or below 600 ml/day, notify the doctor. Also, instruct the patient to follow a diet low in phosphorus.

If serum phosphate levels are decreased, assess the patient for signs and symptoms of hypophosphatemia, such as muscle and bone pain. Have him follow a diet high in phosphorus and avoid antacids containing aluminum hydroxide because they bind with phosphorus. Administer phosphate replacement therapy, as ordered. If I.V. phosphate therapy is prescribed, assess the patient for signs of hypocalcemia, hypokalemia, renal damage, and shock.

Platelet count

Platelets, or thrombocytes, are the smallest formed elements in the blood. Vital to the formation of the homeostatic plug in vascular injury, platelets promote coagulation by supplying phospholipids to the intrinsic thromboplastin pathway.

The platelet count is one of the most important screening tests for platelet function.

Purpose
• To evaluate platelet production

• To assess the effects of chemotherapy or radiation therapy on platelet production

• To aid the diagnoses of thrombocytopenia and thrombocytosis

• To confirm a visual estimate of platelet number and morphology from a stained blood film.

Procedure-related nursing care

Explain the purpose of the test to the patient, and tell him it requires a blood sample.

Perform a venipuncture, collecting the sample in a 7-ml lavender-top tube. Gently mix the sample and the anticoagulant.

Reference values

Normal platelet counts range from 130,000 to 370,000/mm³ (130 to 370 $\times$ 10⁹/L).

Abnormal results

An increased platelet count (thrombocytosis) can result from hemorrhage; infectious disorders; cancer; iron deficiency anemia; recent surgery, pregnancy, or splenectomy; and inflammatory disorders, such as collagen vascular disease. In such cases, the patient's platelet count will return to normal after the patient recovers. However, the platelet count will remain elevated in primary thrombocytosis, myelofibrosis with myeloid metaplasia, polycythemia vera, and chronic myelogenous leukemia.

A decreased platelet count (thrombocytopenia) can result from aplastic or hypoplastic bone marrow disease; infiltrative bone marrow disease, such as carcinoma, leukemia, or disseminated infection; megakaryocytic hypoplasia; ineffective thrombopoiesis caused by folic acid or vitamin B₁₂ deficiency; pooling of platelets in an enlarged spleen; increased platelet destruction caused

by drugs or immune disorders; disseminated intravascular coagulation; Bernard-Soulier syndrome; mechanical injury to platelets; and suppression of bone marrow function caused by chemotherapy or radiation therapy.

Nursing implications of abnormal results

When the platelet count is abnormal, anticipate further studies, such as a complete blood count, bone marrow biopsy, direct antiglobulin test (direct Coombs' test), and serum protein electrophoresis, to establish a diagnosis.

If the patient has a decreased platelet count—especially one that falls below 50,000/mm³—observe him for spontaneous bleeding. Instruct the patient about the importance of protecting himself from injury and reporting any bleeding immediately. And if the count drops below 5,000/mm³, be aware of the risk of fatal central nervous system bleeding or massive GI hemorrhage.

Potassium, serum

This test, a quantitative analysis, measures serum levels of potassium—the major intracellular cation. Vital to homeostasis, potassium maintains cellular osmotic equilibrium. It also helps regulate muscle activity by maintaining electrical conduction within the cardiac and skeletal muscles. As well, potassium helps regulate enzyme activity and acid-base balance and influences kidney function.

Potassium levels are affected by variations in the secretion of adrenal steroid hormones and by fluctuations in pH, serum glucose levels,

Urine potassium test

A quantitative measurement of potassium in the urine, this test evaluates hypokalemia when a health history and physical examination fail to uncover the cause.

Within the body, potassium is filtered through the glomeruli and absorbed through the tubules. For adequate potassium excretion, the distal tubules and collecting ducts must secrete potassium into the urine. By measuring urine potassium levels, it's possible to determine if hypokalemia results from renal disorders, such as renal tubular acidosis, or an extrarenal disorder, such as malabsorption syndrome. The urine potassium test may also aid in the evaluation of renal disease.

Procedure-related nursing care
Collect a 24-hour urine specimen. Refrigerate it or place it on ice during the collection period. At the end of the 24-hour period, send the specimen to the laboratory immediately or put it in the refrigerator until it can be transported.

Reference values
Normal potassium excretion is 25 to 125 mEq/24 hours (25 to 125 mmol/d), with an average potassium concentration of 25 to 100 mEq/liter (25 to 100 mmol/L).

Abnormal results
Renal failure causes decreased urinary excretion of potassium. In a patient with hypokalemia and normal kidney function, urine potassium concentration will be < 10 mEq/liter (< 10 mmol/L), indicating that potassium loss is probably the result of a GI disorder, such as malabsorption syndrome. Hypokalemia lasting more than 3 days and a urine potassium level > 10 mEq/liter indicates a renal loss of potassium that results from aldosteronism, renal tubular acidosis, or Cushing's syndrome.

and serum sodium levels. A reciprocal relationship appears to exist between potassium and sodium; a substantial intake of one element causes a corresponding decrease of the other.

Although the body readily conserves sodium, it has no efficient method for conserving potassium. Even in potassium depletion, the kidneys continue to excrete potassium; therefore, potassium deficiency develops readily and commonly. (See *Urine potassium test.*) Because the kidneys excrete daily nearly all the ingested potassium, a dietary intake of at least 40 mEq/day (40 mmol/d) is essential. (A normal diet usually includes 60 to 100 mEq/day [60 to 100 mmol/d] of potassium.)

Purpose
• To evaluate clinical signs of potassium excess (hyperkalemia) or potassium depletion (hypokalemia)
• To monitor renal function, acid-base balance, and glucose metabolism
• To evaluate neuromuscular and endocrine disorders
• To detect the origin of arrhythmias.

Procedure-related nursing care
Explain the purpose of the test to the patient, and tell him it requires a blood sample. After applying a tourniquet, perform the venipuncture immediately — a delay may elevate the potassium level by allowing intracellular potassium to leak into the serum. Similarly, don't have the

patient make a fist because this can raise the potassium level by 1 mEq/liter or more. Collect the sample in a 10- to 15-ml red-top tube.

Reference values
Normally, serum potassium levels range from 3.8 to 5 mEq/liter (3.8 to 5 mmol/L).

Abnormal results
Abnormally high serum potassium levels are common in patients with burns, crushing injuries, diabetic ketoacidosis, and myocardial infarction — conditions in which excessive cellular potassium enters the blood. Hyperkalemia may also indicate reduced sodium excretion, possibly because of renal failure (preventing normal sodium-potassium exchange) or Addison's disease (caused by the absence of aldosterone, with consequent potassium buildup and sodium depletion).

Decreased potassium values commonly result from aldosteronism or Cushing's syndrome (marked by hypersecretion of adrenal steroid hormones), loss of body fluids (as in diuretic therapy), or excessive licorice ingestion (because of the aldosterone-like effect of glycyrrhizic acid).

Nursing implications of abnormal results
Although serum values and clinical symptoms can indicate a potassium imbalance, check the electrocardiogram (ECG) because it provides the definitive diagnosis.

Observe the patient with elevated serum potassium levels for weakness, malaise, nausea, diarrhea, colicky pain, oliguria, bradycardia, and muscle irritability progressing to flaccid paralysis. The ECG will reveal a prolonged PR interval; a wide QRS complex; a tall, tented T wave;

and ST segment depression.

Report levels greater than 5 mEq/liter and administer medication to reduce potassium levels, as ordered. Dialysis may be needed for a patient with renal failure.

Observe a patient with decreased serum potassium levels for signs of hypokalemia: decreased reflexes; rapid, weak, irregular pulse; mental confusion; hypotension; anorexia; muscle weakness; and paresthesia. In hypokalemia, the ECG will show a flattened T wave, ST segment depression, and U wave elevation. In severe cases, ventricular fibrillation, respiratory paralysis, and cardiac arrest may develop.

If a patient receiving digitalis has a low serum potassium level, watch for signs of digitalis toxicity because the low potassium level enhances the drug's action. Such signs include nausea, vomiting, and bradycardia.

In severe cases of reduced serum potassium levels, administer I.V. potassium chloride (KCl), as ordered. Infuse it at a rate no faster than 20 mEq/hour and at a concentration of no more than 80 mEq/liter of I.V. fluid. Mix the solution well and never give a bolus of KCl because cardiac arrest can occur.

Instruct a patient with low serum potassium levels to eat and drink foods rich in potassium, such as meats, vegetables, fruits, fruit juices, milk, and cola. Also, advise him to take oral potassium preparations, as ordered.

Protein electrophoresis, serum

This test measures serum levels of albumin and globulins, the major

Urine protein test

A quantitative test for proteinuria, a urine protein test aids in the diagnosis of renal disease. Normally, the glomerular membrane allows only proteins of low molecular weight to enter the filtrate. The renal tubules then reabsorb most of these proteins, normally excreting a small amount that's undetectable by a screening test. However, with a damaged glomerular capillary membrane and impaired tubular reabsorption, there will be detectable amounts of proteins excreted in the urine.

A qualitative screening test — a simple dipstick test performed on a random urine sample — is commonly done first. If it's positive, the quantitative analysis of a 24-hour urine specimen by acid precipitation will follow. Electrophoresis can detect Bence-Jones protein, hemoglobins, myoglobins, or albumin in the urine.

Procedure-related nursing care
Collect a 24-hour urine specimen using a special specimen container obtained from the laboratory. Refrigerate the specimen or place it on ice during the collection period. After collecting the entire specimen, transport it to the laboratory immediately.

Reference values
Normally, up to 150 mg of protein will be excreted in 24 hours.

Abnormal results
Heavy proteinuria (more than 4 g/24 hours) is commonly associated with nephrotic syndrome.

Moderate proteinuria (0.5 to 4 g/24 hours) occurs in several types of renal disease — acute or chronic glomerulonephritis, amyloidosis, toxic nephropathies — and in diseases in which renal failure commonly develops as a late complication of the disease, such as diabetes or heart failure.

Minimal proteinuria is most commonly associated with renal diseases in which glomerular involvement isn't a major factor, such as chronic pyelonephritis.

When accompanied by an elevated white blood cell count, proteinuria indicates urinary tract infection; with hematuria, proteinuria indicates local or diffuse urinary tract disorders.

Not all forms of proteinuria have pathologic significance. Benign proteinuria can result from changes in body position. Functional proteinuria is associated with emotional or physiologic stress and is usually transient.

blood proteins, in an electric field by separating the proteins according to their size, shape, and electrical charge at pH 8.6. (Also see *Urine protein test*.) Because each protein fraction moves at a different rate, this movement separates the fractions into recognizable and measurable patterns.

Albumin, which accounts for more than 50% of total serum protein levels, maintains oncotic pressure (preventing capillary plasma leaks) and transports substances that are insoluble in water alone — such as bilirubin, fatty acids, hormones, and drugs.

Four types of globulins exist: alpha$_1$, alpha$_2$, beta, and gamma. The first three types act primarily as carrier proteins that transport lipids, hormones, and metals through the blood. The fourth type, gamma globulin, acts as an important component of the body's immune system.

Although electrophoresis is the most current method for measuring serum protein levels, determinations of total protein and the albumin-

Clinical implications of abnormal protein levels

Abnormal levels of total protein, albumin, or globulin may indicate the following disorders.

INCREASED LEVELS

Total protein
☐ Chronic inflammatory disease (such as rheumatoid arthritis or early stage Laënnec's cirrhosis)
☐ Dehydration
☐ Diabetic acidosis
☐ Fulminating and chronic infections
☐ Monocytic leukemia
☐ Multiple myeloma

Albumin
☐ Multiple myeloma

Globulins
Alpha₁ (α₁)
☐ Acute infections
☐ Cancer
☐ Pregnancy
☐ Tissue necrosis
Alpha₂ (α₂)
☐ Acute infections
☐ Acute myocardial infarction
☐ Advanced cancer
☐ Nephrotic syndrome
☐ Rheumatic fever
☐ Rheumatoid arthritis
☐ Trauma, burns
Beta (β)
☐ Biliary cirrhosis
☐ Cushing's disease
☐ Diabetes mellitus
☐ Hypothyroidism
☐ Malignant hypertension
☐ Nephrotic syndrome
Gamma (γ)
☐ Chronic active liver disease
☐ Hodgkin's disease
☐ Rheumatoid arthritis
☐ Systemic lupus erythematosus

DECREASED LEVELS

Total protein
☐ Benzene and carbon tetrachloride poisoning
☐ Blood dyscrasias
☐ Congestive heart failure
☐ Essential hypertension
☐ GI disease
☐ Hemorrhage
☐ Hepatic dysfunction
☐ Hodgkin's disease
☐ Hyperthyroidism
☐ Malabsorption
☐ Malnutrition
☐ Nephroses
☐ Severe burns
☐ Surgical and traumatic shock
☐ Toxemia of pregnancy
☐ Uncontrolled diabetes mellitus

Albumin
☐ Acute cholecystitis
☐ Collagen diseases
☐ Essential hypertension
☐ Hepatic disease
☐ Hodgkin's disease
☐ Hyperthyroidism
☐ Hypogammaglobulinemia
☐ Malnutrition
☐ Metastatic carcinoma
☐ Nephritis or nephrosis
☐ Peptic ulcer
☐ Plasma loss from burns
☐ Rheumatoid arthritis
☐ Sarcoidosis
☐ Systemic lupus erythematosus

Globulins
Alpha₁ (α₁)
☐ Genetic deficiency of alpha₁-antitrypsin
Alpha₂ (α₂)
☐ Hemolytic anemia
☐ Severe liver disease
Beta (β)
☐ Hypocholesterolemia
Gamma (γ)
☐ Lymphocytic leukemia
☐ Lymphosarcoma
☐ Nephrotic syndrome

globulin (A-G) ratio (normally greater than one) are still commonly performed. No matter which test method is used, a single protein fraction is rarely significant by itself.

Purpose
• To aid the diagnosis of hepatic disease, protein deficiency, blood dyscrasias, renal disorders, and GI and neoplastic diseases.

Procedure-related nursing care
Explain the purpose of the test to the patient, and tell him that it requires a blood sample.

Perform a venipuncture and collect the sample in a 7-ml red-top tube.

Reference values
Values normally fall in these ranges:
• total serum protein levels, 6.6 to 7.9 g/dl (66 to 79 g/L)
• albumin fraction, 3.3 to 4.5 g/dl (33 to 45 g/L)
• alpha$_1$ globulin, 0.1 to 0.4 g/dl (1 to 4 g/L).
• alpha$_2$ globulin, 0.5 to 1 g/dl (5 to 10 g/L)
• beta globulin, 0.7 to 1.2 g/dl (7 to 12 g/L)
• gamma globulin, 0.5 to 1.6 g/dl (5 to 16 g/L).

Abnormal results
Abnormal levels of albumin or globulins are characteristic in many disorders (see *Clinical implications of abnormal protein levels,* page 61).

The A-G ratio is usually evaluated in relation to the total protein level. A low total protein level with a reversed A-G ratio (decreased albumin and elevated globulins) suggests chronic liver disease. A normal total protein level with a reversed A-G ratio suggests myeloproliferative disease (leukemia, Hodgkin's disease) or certain chronic infectious diseases (tuberculosis, chronic hepatitis).

Nursing implications of abnormal results
If the patient's albumin level is decreased, assess him for edema and encourage a high-protein diet, unless the patient has liver disease. If immediate replacement therapy is needed, administer I.V. albumin slowly, as ordered.

If gamma globulin results are abnormal, take appropriate precautions and teach the patient how to protect himself from infection.

Prothrombin time

This test measures the time required for a fibrin clot to form in a citrated plasma sample after calcium ions and tissue thromboplastin (Factor III) have been added. This prothrombin time (PT) is then compared with the fibrin clotting time in a control sample of plasma. The most accurate test results state both the patient's and the control sample's clotting times in seconds.

Because the test reaction bypasses the extrinsic coagulation pathway and doesn't involve the platelets, the test indirectly measures prothrombin activity and is used to evaluate the extrinsic coagulation system, including Factors V, VII, and X, as well as prothrombin and fibrinogen.

The PT test is also the test of choice for monitoring a patient's response to oral anticoagulant therapy.

Purpose
• To monitor a patient's response to

oral anticoagulant therapy
• To evaluate the extrinsic coagulation system
• To aid the diagnosis of conditions associated with abnormal bleeding
• To identify patients at risk for excessive bleeding during surgical or other invasive procedures
• To differentiate deficiencies of specific clotting factors
• To monitor the effects of certain diseases (hepatic disease or protein deficiency, for example) on hemostasis.

Procedure-related nursing care

Explain the purpose of the test to the patient. Tell him it requires a blood sample. If the test is being done to monitor the effects of anticoagulant medications, explain that it will be done daily when therapy begins and will be repeated at longer intervals when medication levels stabilize.

Perform a venipuncture, avoiding excessive probing. Collect the sample in a 7-ml blue-top tube and send it to the laboratory promptly. If transport is delayed more than 4 hours and the sample is kept at room temperature, Factor V may deteriorate, prolonging PT; if the sample is refrigerated, Factor VII may be activated, shortening PT.

Reference values

PT values normally range from 9.6 to 11.8 seconds in men and from 9.5 to 11.3 seconds in women. However, values vary, depending on the source of tissue thromboplastin and the type of sensing devices used to measure clot formation.

Abnormal results

Prolonged PT may indicate deficiencies in fibrinogen, prothrombin, or Factors V, VII, or X (specific assays can pinpoint such deficiencies); vita-

min K deficiency; and hepatic disease. The prolonged time may also result from oral anticoagulant therapy. A prolonged PT that exceeds 2½ times the control value is commonly associated with abnormal bleeding.

Nursing implications of abnormal results

Monitor the PT of patients who are receiving oral anticoagulant therapy. PT is usually maintained between 1½ and 2 times the normal control value. Notify the doctor of results according to policy or as ordered, so he can adjust the medication.

With an increased PT, observe the patient for signs and symptoms of bleeding, such as hematuria, nosebleeds, blood-streaked or tarry stools, hematemesis, and purpura. Keep in mind that when the PT exceeds 40 seconds, bleeding is more apt to occur.

Red blood cell count

Part of a complete blood count, this test determines the number of red blood cells (RBCs) in a cubic millimeter (microliter) of whole blood. An aid in diagnosing anemia and polycythemia, the RBC count (also called the erythrocyte count) doesn't provide qualitative information on the size or shape of RBCs or the weight or concentration of hemoglobin within the RBCs. But the test can be used to calculate two RBC indices, mean corpuscular volume (MCV) and mean corpuscular hemoglobin (MCH). (See *Red blood cell indices,* page 64.)

Purpose

• To supply figures for computing

Red blood cell indices

Red blood cell (RBC) indices help in diagnosing and classifying anemias. Based on the results of the RBC count, hematocrit, and total hemoglobin tests, the indices provide important information about the size of RBCs and the hemoglobin concentration and weight of an average RBC.

The first index, the mean corpuscular volume (MCV) — a ratio of hematocrit, or packed cell volume, to RBC — gives average RBC size. The mean corpuscular hemoglobin (MCH), the ratio of hemoglobin to RBC, expresses the weight of hemoglobin in an average RBC. And the mean corpuscular hemoglobin concentration (MCHC), a ratio of hemoglobin weight to hematocrit, provides the concentration of hemoglobin in 100 ml of packed RBCs.

Procedure-related nursing care
Check for factors that may alter test results. A high white blood cell count, for instance, will falsely elevate the RBC count when automated or semi-automated counters are used, invalidating all test results.

Reference values
Normal MCV ranges from 84 to 99 μ^3/RBC; normal MCH, from 26 to 34 pg/RBC; and normal MCHC, from 30% to 36%.

Abnormal results
A high MCV suggests macrocytic anemias caused by megaloblastic anemias from folic acid or vitamin B_{12} deficiency, inherited disorders of DNA synthesis, or reticulocytosis. Decreased MCV and MCHC indicate microcytic, hypochromic anemias caused by iron deficiency anemia, pyridoxine-responsive anemia, or thalassemia.

• To aid in diagnosis of anemia and polycythemia.

Procedure-related nursing care
Explain the test's purpose to the patient, and tell him you'll need a blood sample. With an infant or a young child, tell the parents that you'll need to draw a small amount of blood — from the heel or great toe of an infant, or the finger or earlobe of a child.

For an adult or older child, draw a venous blood sample, using a 7-ml lavender-top tube. For an infant or a young child, collect a capillary blood sample in a pipette or microcapillary tube. For all patients, fill the collection tube completely, and invert it gently several times to mix the sample and the anticoagulant. Handle the sample gently to prevent hemolysis.

Reference values
RBC values vary according to age, sex, the type of blood sample, and altitude. In men, normal RBC counts range from 4.5 to 6.2 million/mm³ (4.5 to 6.2 × 10¹²/L) of venous blood; in women, from 4.2 to 5.4 million/mm³ (4.2 to 5.4 × 10¹²/L).

In children, normal values range from 4.6 to 4.8 million/mm³ (4.6 to 4.8 × 10¹²/L). For a full-term infant at birth, the normal range extends from 4.4 to 5.8 million/mm³ (4.4 to 5.8 × 10¹²/L) of capillary blood. At age 2 months, the range falls to between 3 and 3.8 million/mm³ (3 and 3.8 × 10¹²/L). Levels slowly increase after age 2 months.

People living at high altitudes usually have higher values.

Abnormal results
An elevated RBC count may indicate primary or secondary polycythemia or dehydration. A depressed count may signify anemia, fluid overload,

the RBC indices, which reveal RBC size and hemoglobin concentration and weight or recent hemorrhage. Further studies, such as stained cell examination, hematocrit, hemoglobin levels, RBC indices, and white blood cell counts, confirm a diagnosis.

Nursing implications of abnormal results

If the patient has an increased RBC count, keep him as active as possible. A rise in RBC levels signals increased blood viscosity, putting him at greater risk for venous thrombi formation.

Make sure he receives enough fluids. If he's NPO, he'll need I.V. fluid replacement.

If the patient has a decreased RBC count, assess him for signs and symptoms of anemia, including fatigue, pallor, dyspnea on exertion, tachycardia, and headache. If a patient has mild anemia, you may not detect any signs and symptoms of the problem.

Emphasize the importance of complying with iron supplement therapy and maintaining an iron-rich diet. Tell the patient to take iron supplements with meals, but not with milk or antacids, which can interfere with iron absorption. Explain to him that the iron supplements may cause his stool to look dark and tarry. Also, teach him to eat iron-rich foods, such as red meat, green vegetables, and iron-fortified bread.

Sodium, serum

The serum sodium test measures the amount of sodium—the major extracellular cation—in the blood. Sodium affects body water distribution, maintains osmotic pressure of extracellular fluid, and helps promote neuromuscular function. So-dium also helps maintain acid-base balance and influences chloride and potassium levels. Sodium is absorbed by the intestines and excreted primarily by the kidneys. A small amount of sodium is lost through the skin.

Extracellular sodium concentration helps the kidneys regulate body water. Decreased sodium levels promote water excretion, and increased levels promote retention. For this reason, serum sodium levels are evaluated in relation to the amount of water in the body. Thus, a sodium deficit (hyponatremia) refers to a decreased level of sodium in relation to the body's water level.

The body normally regulates this sodium-water balance through aldosterone, which inhibits sodium excretion and promotes its resorption (with water) by the renal tubules. Decreased sodium levels stimulate aldosterone secretion, and elevated sodium levels depress aldosterone secretion.

Purpose
- To evaluate fluid-electrolyte and acid-base balance and related neuromuscular, renal, and adrenal functions
- To evaluate the effects of drug therapy (such as diuretics) on serum sodium levels.

Procedure-related nursing care
Explain the purpose of the test to the patient. Tell him it requires a blood sample.

Perform a venipuncture, collecting the sample in a 10- to 15-ml red-top tube. Handle the sample gently because hemolysis may affect test results.

Reference values
Serum levels of sodium normally range between 135 and 145 mEq/

Urine sodium test

This test, which determines urine levels of sodium, is commonly performed in conjunction with urine chloride tests. Less significant than serum levels — and consequently, performed less frequently — the urine sodium test evaluates renal conservation of sodium and chloride and confirms serum sodium values. Normally, when the serum sodium level is high, renal excretion of sodium increases; when the serum sodium level is low, the kidneys conserve sodium.

Reference values
Normal urine sodium excretion is 30 to 280 mEq/24 hours (30 to 280 mmol/d); the amount varies greatly with dietary salt intake and perspiration.

Abnormal results
Increased urine sodium levels are associated with renal tubular dysfunction because this condition affects sodium reabsorption. It occurs in such disorders as chronic pyelonephritis and acute tubular necrosis. Other causes of increased urine sodium levels include diabetic acidosis and Addison's disease.

With a decreased glomerular filtration rate, as occurs in glomerulonephritis, the urine sodium level decreases. Other causes of a decrease include congestive heart failure and Cushing's disease.

Nursing considerations
Expect urine sodium and urine chloride levels to be parallel, rising and falling in tandem.

Remember that urine sodium levels should be correlated with the results of serum electrolyte studies when you're evaluating a fluid-electrolyte imbalance.

---

liter (135 and 145 mmol/L).

Abnormal results
Elevated serum sodium levels (hypernatremia) may result from inadequate water intake, water loss that exceeds sodium loss (as in diabetes insipidus, impaired renal function, and prolonged hyperventilation), and sodium retention (as in aldosteronism). Hypernatremia can also result from excessive sodium intake.

Hyponatremia may result from inadequate sodium intake or excessive sodium loss caused by profuse sweating, GI suctioning, diuretic therapy, diarrhea, vomiting, adrenal insufficiency, burns, or chronic renal insufficiency with acidosis.

Nursing implications of abnormal results
Serum sodium levels must be interpreted in light of the patient's state of hydration. In some cases, you may evaluate serum sodium levels along with the results of a urine sodium test. Many times, urine sodium levels are more sensitive to early changes in sodium balance. (See *Urine sodium test*.)

Increased sodium levels. Observe a patient with hypernatremia associated with water loss for thirst, restlessness, dry and sticky mucous membranes, flushed skin, oliguria, and diminished reflexes. However, if an increased total body sodium level causes water retention, observe for hypertension, dyspnea, and edema. Teach the patient to avoid foods high in sodium — such as corned beef, bacon, ham, canned or smoked fish, cheese, celery, condiments, canned vegetables, olives, potato chips, and cola drinks. Tell him to avoid using salt when cooking and eating.

Keep an accurate record of intake and output, and weigh the patient daily to check for body fluid loss.

Check urine specific gravity. A specific gravity over 1.030 can occur with hypernatremia.

Decreased sodium levels. Watch a patient with hyponatremia for apprehension, lassitude, headache, decreased skin turgor, abdominal cramps, and a tremor that may progress to seizures. Encourage him to drink fluids with solutes, such as fruit juices and broth.

Irrigate nasogastric tubes with normal saline solution instead of sterile water.

Check urine specific gravity; results less than 1.010 are likely to occur in hyponatremia.

Triglycerides, serum

This test provides a quantitative analysis of triglycerides—the main storage form of lipids. Triglycerides consist of one molecule of glycerol bonded to three molecules of fatty acids. Thus, the degradation of triglycerides leads directly to the production of fatty acids. Together with carbohydrates, triglycerides furnish energy for metabolism.

Triglyceride testing shouldn't be performed while a patient is hospitalized for a myocardial infarction because this condition causes an increase in very-low-density lipoproteins and a decrease in low-density lipoproteins.

Purpose
• To determine the risk of coronary artery disease (CAD)
• To screen for hyperlipemia
• To identify disorders associated with altered triglyceride levels.

Procedure-related nursing care
Explain the purpose of the test to the patient, and tell him it requires a blood sample. Instruct him to abstain from alcohol for 24 hours before the test and from food for 12 to 14 hours before the test. Also tell him not to take any medications, such as corticosteroids, that may alter his test results.

Perform a venipuncture and collect the sample in a 7-ml red-top tube.

After the test, tell the patient he can resume his normal diet.

Reference values
Triglyceride values are age-related. Some controversy exists over the most appropriate normal ranges, but the following are fairly well accepted:
• ages 0 to 29: 10 to 140 mg/dl (0.1 to 1.55 mmol/L)
• ages 30 to 39: 10 to 150 mg/dl (0.1 to 1.65 mmol/L)
• ages 40 to 49: 10 to 160 mg/dl (0.1 to 1.75 mmol/L)
• ages 50 to 59: 10 to 190 mg/dl (0.1 to 2.1 mmol/L).

Abnormal results
Increased or decreased serum triglyceride levels suggest a clinical abnormality that requires additional testing, such as cholesterol measurement, for a definitive diagnosis.

High levels of triglycerides and cholesterol reflect an increased risk of atherosclerosis or CAD.

Markedly increased levels without an identifiable cause reflect congenital hyperlipoproteinemia and require lipoprotein phenotyping to confirm the diagnosis.

A mild to moderate increase in serum triglyceride levels indicates biliary obstruction, diabetes, nephrotic syndrome, endocrinopathies, or excessive consumption of alcohol.

Decreased serum levels are rare, occurring mainly in malnutrition or abetalipoproteinemia.

Nursing implications of abnormal results

Expect a lipoprotein electrophoresis or a serum cholesterol test to be ordered for the patient with an increased serum triglyceride level. Teach him to avoid eating large amounts of sugars, carbohydrates, and dietary fats. Encourage him to eat fruit.

Uric acid, serum

Used primarily to detect gout, this test measures serum levels of uric acid—the major end metabolite of purine. Large amounts of purines are present in nucleic acids and are derived from dietary and endogenous sources. Uric acid clears the body by glomerular filtration and tubular secretion. (See *Urine uric acid test*.)

Purpose
• To confirm a diagnosis of gout
• To help detect kidney dysfunction.

Urine uric acid test

A quantitative analysis of uric acid levels in the urine, this test supplements serum uric acid testing by measuring the efficiency of renal uric acid clearance. It helps identify disorders that alter production or excretion of uric acid, such as leukemia, gout, and renal dysfunction. As the chief end product of purine catabolism, uric acid passes from the liver through the bloodstream to the kidneys, where roughly 50% is excreted daily in the urine. The test requires collection of a 24-hour urine specimen.

Reference values
Normal uric acid values in the urine vary with diet but generally range between 250 and 750 mg/24 hours (1.5 to 4.5 mmol/d).

Abnormal results
Elevated urine uric acid levels may result from chronic myeloid leukemia, polycythemia vera, multiple myeloma, and early remission in pernicious anemia, as well as lymphosarcoma and lymphatic leukemia during radiotherapy. High levels also result from tubular reabsorption defects, such as Fanconi's syndrome and hepatolenticular degeneration (Wilson's disease).

Low urine uric acid levels occur in gout (when associated with normal uric acid production but inadequate excretion) and with severe renal damage, such as that resulting from chronic glomerulonephritis, diabetic glomerulosclerosis, and collagen disorders.

Nursing considerations
Be aware that diuretics can decrease uric acid excretion. Low doses of salicylates, phenylbutazone, and probenecid also lower urine uric acid levels; high doses of these drugs cause levels to rise above normal. Allopurinol, a drug used to treat gout, increases uric acid excretion.

Expect uric acid concentrations to rise with a high-purine diet and fall with a low-purine diet.

Procedure-related nursing care

Explain the purpose of the test to the patient. Tell him it requires a blood sample.

Perform a venipuncture and collect the sample in a 10- to 15-ml red-top tube. Handle the sample gently to prevent hemolysis.

Reference values

Uric acid concentrations in men normally range from 4.3 to 8 mg/dl (260 to 480 µmol/L); in women, from 2.3 to 6 mg/dl (140 to 360 µmol/L).

Abnormal results

Increased serum uric acid levels usually indicate impaired renal function or gout. However, in gout, levels don't correlate with the severity of the disease. Levels also may rise in congestive heart failure, glycogen storage disease (type I, von Gierke's disease), acute infectious diseases (such as infectious mononucleosis), hemolytic or sickle cell anemia, hemoglobinopathies, polycythemia, leukemia, lymphoma, metastatic cancer, and psoriasis.

Depressed serum uric acid levels may indicate defective renal tubular reabsorption (as in Fanconi's syndrome and Wilson's disease) or acute hepatic atrophy.

Nursing implications of abnormal results

If the patient has an increased serum uric acid level, teach him to avoid eating foods high in purine (see *Foods with purine*). If appropriate, explain the need to decrease alcohol consumption because alcohol can cause renal retention of uric acid. Also observe the patient for signs and symptoms of gout, such as swollen, painful joints.

If the patient's serum uric acid level is elevated and his urine output is decreased, anticipate tests for serum urea and serum creatinine levels.

Foods with purine

The patient with a high serum level of uric acid should try to avoid these foods containing purine nitrogen.

High amounts	Moderate amounts
☐ Organ meats	☐ Meat
☐ Sweetbreads	☐ Poultry
☐ Roe	☐ Shellfish
☐ Sardines	☐ Asparagus
☐ Scallops	☐ Beans
☐ Mackerel	☐ Mushrooms
☐ Anchovies	☐ Peas
☐ Broth, consommé	☐ Spinach

Urinalysis, routine

A common test, routine urinalysis is used to screen for urinary and systemic disorders. Abnormal findings suggest disease and indicate the need for further urine or blood tests to identify the problem.

Laboratory methods for detecting or measuring urine components include the evaluation of physical characteristics, such as color, odor, and opacity; screening for pH, protein, sugars, and ketone bodies; refractometry for measuring specific gravity; and microscopic inspection of centrifuged sediment for cells, casts, and crystals.

Purpose

● To screen for renal or urinary tract disease

Normal results in routine urinalysis

ELEMENT	RESULT
Macroscopic	
Color	Straw
Odor	Slightly aromatic
Appearance	Clear
Specific gravity	1.005 to 1.020
pH	4.5 to 8.0
Protein	None
Glucose	None
Ketones	None
Other sugars	None
Microscopic	
Red blood cells	0 to 3/high-power field
White blood cells	0 to 4/high-power field
Epithelial cells	Few
Casts	None, except occasional hyaline casts
Crystals	Few
Yeast cells	None
Parasites	None

● To help detect metabolic or systemic disease.

Procedure-related nursing care

Explain the test's purpose to the patient. Tell him to avoid strenuous exercise before the test because it may cause transient myoglobinuria and inaccurate results. Obtain a dietary history. Excessive amounts of foods such as carrots, rhubarb, and beets may cause a change in urine color, and excessive amounts of foods such as meats and cranberry juice can lower pH.

Collect a clean-catch urine specimen of at least 15 ml. If possible, obtain a first-voided morning specimen because it contains the greatest concentration of solutes. If the urine appears concentrated or dilute, assess the patient's fluid status — dehydration and a decreased or increased fluid intake can affect the urine.

Send the specimen to the laboratory immediately, or refrigerate it if analysis will be delayed longer than 1 hour.

Normal results

A routine urinalysis includes a macroscopic and microscopic evaluation (see *Normal results in routine urinalysis*).

Abnormal results

The following abnormal results generally suggest pathologic conditions.

Color. Changes in color can result from diet, drugs, and many metabolic, inflammatory, and infectious diseases.

Odor. In diabetes mellitus, starvation, and dehydration, a fruity odor accompanies formation of ketone bodies. In urinary tract infection (UTI), a fetid odor is common, especially if *Escherichia coli* is present. Maple syrup urine disease and phenylketonuria also cause distinctive odors.

Turbidity. Turbid urine may contain red blood cells (RBCs), white blood cells (WBCs), bacteria, fat, or chyle and may reflect renal infection.

Specific gravity. Low specific gravity

(less than 1.005) is characteristic of diabetes insipidus, nephrogenic diabetes insipidus, acute tubular necrosis, and pyelonephritis. Fixed specific gravity, in which values remain 1.010 regardless of fluid intake, occurs in chronic glomerulonephritis with severe renal damage. High specific gravity (greater than 1.020) occurs in nephrotic syndrome, dehydration, acute glomerulonephritis, congestive heart failure, liver failure, and shock.

pH. Alkaline urine pH may result from Fanconi's syndrome, UTI, and metabolic or respiratory alkalosis. Acid urine pH is associated with renal tuberculosis, pyrexia, phenylketonuria, alkaptonuria, and all forms of acidosis.

Protein. Proteinuria suggests renal diseases, such as nephrosis, glomerulosclerosis, glomerulonephritis, nephrolithiasis, polycystic kidney disease, and renal failure. Proteinuria can also result from multiple myeloma.

Sugars. Glycosuria usually indicates diabetes mellitus but may also result from pheochromocytoma, Cushing's syndrome, and increased intracranial pressure. Fructosuria, galactosuria, and pentosuria generally suggest rare hereditary metabolic disorders. However, an alimentary form of pentosuria and fructosuria may follow excessive ingestion of pentose or fructose, resulting in hepatic failure to metabolize the sugar. Since the renal tubules fail to reabsorb pentose or fructose, these sugars spill over into the urine.

Ketones. Ketonuria occurs in diabetes mellitus when cellular energy needs exceed the available cellular glucose. In the absence of glucose, cells will metabolize fat, an alternate energy supply. Ketone bodies—the end products of incomplete fat metabolism—accumulate in plasma and are excreted in the urine. Ketonuria may also occur in starvation states and in conditions of acutely increased metabolic demand associated with decreased food intake, such as diarrhea or vomiting.

Cells. Hematuria indicates bleeding within the genitourinary tract and may result from infection, obstruction, inflammation, trauma, tumors, glomerulonephritis, renal hypertension, lupus nephritis, renal tuberculosis, renal vein thrombosis, hydronephrosis, pyelonephritis, scurvy, malaria, parasitic infection of the bladder, subacute bacterial endocarditis, polyarteritis nodosa, and hemorrhagic disorders. Numerous WBCs in urine usually imply urinary tract inflammation, especially cystitis or pyelonephritis. WBCs and WBC casts in urine suggest renal infection. An excessive number of epithelial cells suggests renal tubular degeneration.

Casts. Plugs of gelled protein, known as casts, form in the renal tubules and collecting ducts by agglutination of protein cells or cellular debris. These casts are flushed loose by urine flow. An excessive number of casts indicates renal disease. Hyaline casts are associated with renal parenchymal disease, inflammation, and trauma to the glomerular capillary membrane; epithelial casts, with renal tubular damage, nephrosis, eclampsia, amyloidosis, and heavy metal poisoning; coarse and fine granular casts, with acute or chronic renal failure, pyelonephritis, and chronic lead intoxication; fatty and waxy casts, with nephrotic syndrome, chronic renal disease, and diabetes mellitus; RBC casts, with renal parenchymal disease (especially glomerulonephritis), renal infarction, subacute bacterial endocarditis, vascular disorders, sickle cell anemia, scurvy, blood dyscrasias, malignant hypertension, collagen disease, and acute inflammation; and WBC casts, with acute pyelonephritis and glomerulonephritis, nephrotic syndrome, pyogenic infection, and lupus nephritis.

Crystals. Some crystals normally appear in urine, but numerous calcium oxalate crystals suggest hypercalcemia. Cystine crystals (cystinuria) reflect an inborn metabolism error.

Other components. Yeast cells and parasites in urine sediment reflect genitourinary tract infection, as well as contamination of external genitalia. Yeast cells, which may be mistaken for RBCs, can be identified by their ovoid shape, lack of color, variable size and, in many cases, signs of budding. The most common parasite in sediment is *Trichomonas vaginalis,* a flagellated protozoan that commonly causes vaginitis, urethritis, and prostatovesiculitis.

Nursing implications of abnormal results
If any of the results are abnormal, anticipate further diagnostic tests.

White blood cell count

Part of the complete blood count, the white blood cell (WBC) count reports the number of WBCs found in a cubic millimeter (microliter) of whole blood. On any given day, the WBC count can vary by as much as 2,000. Such variations may result from strenuous exercise, stress, or digestion. The WBC count can rise or fall significantly in certain diseases, but the count is diagnostically useful only when interpreted in light of the WBC differential and the patient's current clinical status.

Purpose
• To determine the presence of infection or inflammation
• To determine the need for further tests, such as the WBC differential or bone marrow biopsy
• To monitor a patient's response to chemotherapy or radiation therapy.

Procedure-related nursing care
Explain the purpose of the test to the patient. Tell him to avoid strenuous exercise for 24 hours before the test and to avoid eating a heavy meal before the test. If he's receiving treatment for an infection, advise him that this test may be repeated to monitor his progress.

Perform a venipuncture, collecting the sample in a 7-ml lavender-top tube. Handle the sample gently to prevent hemolysis.

After the procedure, tell the patient he may resume normal activities.

Reference values
The WBC count ranges from 4,100 to 10,900/mm³ (4.1 to 10.9 × 10⁹/L).

Abnormal results
An elevated WBC count (leukocytosis) usually signals infection. A high count may also result from leukemia and tissue necrosis caused by burns, myocardial infarction, or gangrene.

A low WBC count (leukopenia) indicates bone marrow depression that can result from viral infections or from toxic reactions after ingestion of mercury or other heavy metals, treatment with antineoplastics, or exposure to benzene or arsenicals. Leukopenia also characteristically accompanies influenza, typhoid fever, measles, infectious hepatitis, mononucleosis, and rubella.

Nursing implications of abnormal results

If the patient has an increased WBC count, ask if he has recently exercised, eaten, or been under stress. Take his vital signs, noting any elevation in temperature or pulse rate. Check for signs and symptoms of inflammation and infection.

If the patient has a decreased WBC count, ask if he's taking any over-the-counter drugs, then ask the pharmacist if they can cause agranulocytosis. Advise a patient with leukopenia to avoid people with contagious conditions because of his reduced resistance to infection.

White blood cell differential

Because the white blood cell (WBC) differential evaluates the distribution and morphology of WBCs, it provides more specific information about a patient's immune function than the WBC count. The differential count represents the relative number of each type of WBC in the blood. Multiplying the percentage value of each type by the total WBC count provides the absolute number of each type of WBC.

Purpose
• To evaluate the body's capacity to resist and overcome infection
• To detect and identify various types of leukemia
• To determine the stage and sever-

Reference values for WBC differential

ADULTS		
CELLS	**RELATIVE VALUE**	**ABSOLUTE VALUE**
Neutrophils	47.6% to 76.8%	1,950 to 8,400/mm^3
Eosinophils	0.3% to 7%	12 to 760/mm^3
Basophils	0.3% to 2%	12 to 200/mm^3
Lymphocytes	16.2% to 43%	660 to 4,600/mm^3
Monocytes	0.6% to 9.6%	24 to 960/mm^3

CHILDREN (ages 6 to 17)		
CELLS	**RELATIVE VALUE (Boys)**	**RELATIVE VALUE (Girls)**
Neutrophils	38.5% to 71.5%	41.9% to 76.5%
Eosinophils	1% to 8.1%	0.8% to 8.3%
Basophils	0.25% to 1.3%	0.3% to 1.4%
Lymphocytes	19.4% to 51.4%	16.3% to 46.7%
Monocytes	1.1% to 11.6%	0.9% to 9.9%

How disease influences the WBC differential count

CELL TYPE	HOW AFFECTED
Neutrophils	**Increased by:** • Infections — osteomyelitis, otitis media, salpingitis, septicemia, gonorrhea, endocarditis, smallpox, chicken pox, herpes, Rocky Mountain spotted fever • Ischemic necrosis from myocardial infarction, burns, carcinoma • Metabolic disorders — diabetic acidosis, eclampsia, uremia, thyrotoxicosis • Stress response from acute hemorrhage, surgery, excessive exercise, emotional distress, third trimester of pregnancy, childbirth • Inflammatory diseases — rheumatic fever, rheumatoid arthritis, acute gout, vasculitis, myositis **Decreased by:** • Bone marrow depression from radiation or cytotoxic drugs • Infections — typhoid, tularemia, brucellosis, hepatitis, influenza, measles, mumps, rubella, infectious mononucleosis • Hypersplenism — hepatic disease and storage diseases • Collagen vascular diseases — systemic lupus erythematosus • Deficiency of folic acid or vitamin B_{12}
Eosinophils	**Increased by:** • Allergic disorders — asthma, hay fever, food or drug sensitivity, serum sickness, angioneurotic edema • Parasitic infections — trichinosis, hookworm, roundworm, amebiasis • Skin diseases — eczema, pemphigus, psoriasis, dermatitis, herpes • Neoplastic diseases — chronic myelocytic leukemia, Hodgkin's disease, metastases and necrosis of solid tumors • Miscellaneous — collagen vascular disease, adrenocortical hypofunction, ulcerative colitis, polyarteritis nodosa, postsplenectomy, pernicious anemia, scarlet fever, excessive exercise **Decreased by:** • Stress response from trauma, shock, burns, surgery, mental distress • Cushing's syndrome
Basophils	**Increased by:** • Miscellaneous — chronic myelocytic leukemia, polycythemia vera, some chronic hemolytic anemias, Hodgkin's disease, systemic mastocytosis, myxedema, ulcerative colitis, chronic hypersensitivity states, nephrosis **Decreased by:** • Miscellaneous — hyperthyroidism, ovulation, pregnancy, stress
Lymphocytes	**Increased by:** • Infections — pertussis, brucellosis, syphilis, tuberculosis, hepatitis, infectious mononucleosis, mumps, German measles, cytomegalovirus • Miscellaneous — thyrotoxicosis, hypoadrenalism, ulcerative colitis, immune diseases, lymphocytic leukemia **Decreased by:** • Severe debilitating illness — congestive heart failure, renal failure, advanced tuberculosis • Miscellaneous — defective lymphatic circulation, high levels of adrenal corticosteroids, immunodeficiency due to immunosuppressives

How disease influences the WBC differential count (continued)

CELL TYPE	HOW AFFECTED
Monocytes	**Increased by:** • Infections — subacute bacterial endocarditis, tuberculosis, hepatitis, malaria, Rocky Mountain spotted fever • Collagen vascular diseases — systemic lupus erythematosus, rheumatoid arthritis, polyarteritis nodosa • Neoplastic diseases — carcinomas, monocytic leukemia, lymphomas

ity of an infection
• To detect allergic reactions
• To assess the severity of allergic reactions (eosinophil count)
• To detect parasitic infections.

Procedure-related nursing care
Explain the purpose of the test to the patient and tell him it requires a blood sample. Instruct him to avoid strenuous exercise for 24 hours before the test.

Perform a venipuncture, collecting the sample in a 7-ml lavender-top tube.

Reference values
Reference values for the five types of WBC differentials — neutrophils, eosinophils, basophils, lymphocytes, and monocytes — are based on whether the patient is an adult or a child (see *Reference values for WBC differential*, page 73).

Abnormal results
Abnormal differential patterns provide evidence of a wide range of conditions. (See *How disease influences the WBC differential count*.)

Nursing implications of abnormal results
Check the WBC differential count when reviewing the WBC count. Ab-

normal levels of specific WBC types may indicate certain disorders. For example, an increased eosinophil level may be a sign of an allergy.

Also assess the patient for conditions associated with specific abnormal WBC results. An increase in basophils, for instance, is associated with the healing process. So in a patient with this test result, you may detect signs of healing, such as decreased amounts of exudate at an infectious site or better movement in an injured extremity.

Suggested readings

Clinical Laboratory Tests: Values and Implications. Springhouse, Pa.: Springhouse Corp., 1991.

Diagnostics, 2nd ed. Nurse's Reference Library. Springhouse, Pa.: Springhouse Corp., 1987.

Kee, J.L. *Handbook of Laboratory and Diagnostic Tests with Nursing Implications.* Norwalk, Conn.: Appleton & Lange, 1990.

Pagana, K.D., and Pagana, T.J. *Diagnostic Testing and Nursing Implications: A Case Study Approach,* 3rd ed. St. Louis: C.V. Mosby Co., 1990.

Speicher, C.E. *The Right Test: A Physician's Guide to Laboratory Medicine.* Philadelphia: W.B. Saunders Co., 1989.

2

CULTURE STUDIES

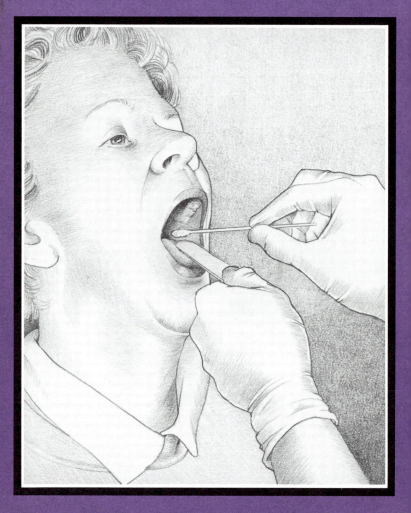

When a doctor suspects that a patient has an infection, he may order a culture study to confirm his suspicion. Such a study can not only isolate and identify the pathogen, but also provide information that helps guide the selection of anti-infective therapy.

For these diagnostic tests, you'll collect the appropriate specimen and, in some cases, place it in an artificial medium (or culture) that allows microorganisms to flourish. You'll then send the culture to the laboratory, where the atmosphere, temperature, and pH will be strictly controlled during incubation.

The length of the incubation depends on such factors as the growth rate and nutritional requirements of the organism. Most common bacterial pathogens can be isolated in 24 to 48 hours. Fungi and microbacteria may take several weeks.

Once a microbe is isolated, its susceptibility to specific anti-infectives and the extent of the patient's infection can be determined. Based on this information, the patient's doctor can select the appropriate anti-infective therapy.

Procedure-related nursing care

The following nursing care measures apply to all culture studies covered in this chapter. As part of the discussion of each culture study, you'll also find specific nursing care considerations.

Before the procedure. Before collecting a specimen for any culture study, explain the procedure to the patient. If he'll be collecting the specimen himself, give him the appropriate container and tell him what he needs to do. If you don't know which collection container to use, you can check your hospital's procedure manual or ask the appropriate laboratory technician.

If possible, postpone any anti-infective therapy until after you've collected the specimen. Previous or current therapy may cause a false-negative culture or delayed growth.

If you'll be performing the procedure, wash your hands thoroughly and put on clean gloves.

During the procedure. Use strict aseptic technique when obtaining the specimen. Also be sure you obtain a sufficient specimen. Repeat cultures cost time and money and may cause the patient unnecessary pain. If you think more than one specimen is necessary — for instance, if the patient has a large wound or multiple infection sites — consult the doctor. If he orders specimens from different sites, use a separate sterile container for each.

Close the container tightly to prevent a spill or contamination. If the patient is in isolation or the container becomes soiled, wipe it with a bactericide before sending it to the laboratory.

After the procedure. Label the container with the patient's name, room number, specimen type, and such specifics as wound location, if applicable; suspected diagnosis; date; and collection time. Number multiple containers in sequential order, and prepare a laboratory slip for each. Note any isolation precautions or anti-infective therapy on the slip and the culture container.

Send the specimen to the laboratory as soon as possible to prevent organism destruction or overgrowth. For a viral culture, pack the container in ice and send it to the laboratory immediately. Certain specimens can be refrigerated briefly if you can't transport them right away. Check with laboratory personnel for the correct procedure.

Properly dispose of your gloves, then wash your hands. Make sure the patient is clean and comfortable. Observe the patient for signs that his condition is improving or worsening.

Nursing implications of abnormal results

If the test confirms an infection, administer anti-infective therapy, as ordered.

Blood culture

For this test, a culture medium is inoculated with a sample of the patient's blood so the pathogens causing bacteremia and septicemia can be isolated and identified. A blood culture can identify about 67% of pathogens within 24 hours and up to 90% within 72 hours.

Bacteria from local tissue infection usually invade the bloodstream through the lymphatic system via the thoracic duct. Occasionally, the bacteria enter the bloodstream directly through infusion lines or as a result of thrombophlebitis or bacterial endocarditis.

Bacteremia may be transient, intermittent, or continuous. The specimen is usually withdrawn before drug therapy begins and when the bacterial count is expected to be high.

Purpose
• To confirm bacteremia
• To identify the organism causing bacteremia and septicemia.

Procedure-related nursing care
Besides performing the nursing care discussed in the chapter introduc-

tion, take the following specific measures. Explain to the patient that the test requires a blood sample. If you'll be obtaining the sample, clean the venipuncture site first with an alcohol swab, then with an iodine swab. Start at the site and work outward in a circular motion. Allow the skin to dry for at least 1 minute after applying the iodine. Then remove the residual iodine with an alcohol swab. Or you can remove the iodine after the venipuncture.

If you're using culture bottles with broth or resin, collect the blood in a syringe. If the lysis-centrifugation technique will be used, collect the blood in a special collection or processing tube. Perform the venipuncture and withdraw 10 to 20 ml of blood for an adult or 2 to 6 ml for a child.

If you're using culture bottles, clean the diaphragm tops with alcohol or iodine swabs and change the needle on the syringe. If you're using broth, add blood to each bottle until you obtain a 1:5 to 1:10 dilution. For example, add 10 ml of blood to a 100-ml bottle. (The size of the bottle will vary according to your hospital's policy.) If you're using a special resin, add equal amounts of blood to the resin in the bottles. Gently invert the bottles to mix the blood and resin.

Send the bottles or the special collection or processing tube to the laboratory immediately.

Normal results
Blood cultures are normally sterile.

Abnormal results
Positive blood cultures don't necessarily confirm septicemia because many organisms may invade the bloodstream temporarily during the early stages of infection. Mild, transient bacteremia may occur during

the course of many infectious diseases or may complicate other disorders. Persistent, continuous, or recurrent bacteremia reliably confirms a serious infection.

Common blood pathogens include *Neisseria meningitidis, Streptococcus pneumoniae* and other *Streptococcus* species, *Haemophilus influenzae, Staphylococcus aureus, Pseudomonas aeruginosa,* Bacteroidaceae, *Brucella*, and Enterobacteriaceae. Although 2% to 3% of the blood samples cultured are contaminated by skin bacteria — such as *Staphylococcus epidermidis* and diphtheroids — these organisms may be clinically significant when isolated from multiple cultures.

Nasopharyngeal culture

This test, an evaluation of nasopharyngeal secretions, is used to identify pathogenic organisms, such as *Bordetella pertussis* and *Neisseria meningitidis* — especially in young, elderly, or debilitated patients. Nasopharyngeal culture can also be used to isolate viruses, especially to identify carriers of influenza A and B viruses. However, testing for viruses is complex, time-consuming, and costly, and thus infrequently done.

Purpose
• To identify pathogens causing upper respiratory tract symptoms
• To identify the proliferation of normal nasopharyngeal flora, which may prove pathogenic in debilitated and other immunologically vulnerable patients
• To identify asymptomatic carriers of infectious organisms, such as *B. pertussis* and *N. meningitidis*.

Obtaining a nasopharyngeal specimen

You can obtain a nasopharyngeal specimen by one of two methods: direct swabbing of the area or swabbing through an open-ended, tempered-glass tube. The former is more common.

For either method, put on gloves and ask the patient to cough. Then position him with his head tilted back. Using a penlight and a tongue blade, inspect the nasopharyngeal area.

Direct swab
Gently pass a sterile, cotton-tipped swab through the nostril and into the nasopharynx, as shown. Keep the swab near the septum and the floor of the nose. To avoid contaminating the specimen, don't touch the sides of the patient's nostril with the swab. Quickly rotate the swab and remove it without injuring the nasal mucous membrane.

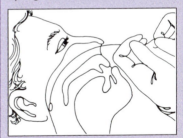

Tempered-glass tube
Place the open-ended, tempered-glass tube in the patient's nostril. Carefully pass the sterile, cotton-tipped swab through the tube and into the nasopharynx. (The tube prevents you from contaminating the specimen with the sides of the patient's nostril.) When the swab reaches the nasopharynx, rotate it gently for 5 seconds. Then remove the swab and place it in the culture tube with a transport medium. Remove the tempered-glass tube.

Procedure-related nursing care

Besides performing the nursing care discussed in the chapter introduction, you'll need to obtain a nasopharyngeal specimen (see *Obtaining a nasopharyngeal specimen*, page 79).

Normal results

Flora normally found in the nasopharynx includes nonhemolytic streptococci, alpha-hemolytic streptococci, *Neisseria* species (except *N. meningitidis* and *N. gonorrhoeae*), coagulase-negative staphylococci such as *Staphylococcus epidermidis* and, occasionally, the coagulase-positive *Staphylococcus aureus*.

Abnormal results

Pathogens that indicate infection include group A beta-hemolytic streptococci; occasionally groups B, C, and G beta-hemolytic streptococci; *B. pertussis*; *Corynebacterium diphtheriae*; *S. aureus*; and large numbers of *Haemophilus influenzae*, pneumococci, or *Candida albicans*.

Sputum culture

A bacteriologic examination of sputum helps identify the cause of a pulmonary infection and guide the treatment for lung disease. The most common method of specimen collection is expectoration. Less common methods include nasotracheal suctioning and bronchoscopy. Nasotracheal suctioning is contraindicated for a patient with esophageal varices or cardiac disease. Only a doctor will perform bronchoscopy to collect a specimen.

Purpose

• To isolate and identify the cause of a pulmonary infection, thus aiding in the diagnosis of respiratory diseases (most frequently bronchitis, tuberculosis, lung abscess, and pneumonia).

Procedure-related nursing care

Besides performing the nursing care discussed in the chapter introduction, you'll need to obtain a sputum specimen. For the expectoration method, instruct the patient to take three deep breaths and cough forcefully, expectorating into the container. Tell him not to spit saliva into the container. If his cough is nonproductive, use chest physiotherapy, a heated aerosol spray, or intermittent positive-pressure breathing with a prescribed aerosol to induce sputum, as ordered.

Using aseptic technique, close the container securely and seal it in a leakproof bag before sending it to the laboratory.

For the nasotracheal suctioning method, see *Obtaining a specimen by nasotracheal suction*.

Normal results

The flora normally found in the respiratory tract includes alpha-hemolytic streptococci, *Neisseria* species, and diphtheroids. The presence of normal flora doesn't rule out an infection.

Abnormal results

Because sputum is invariably contaminated with normal oropharyngeal flora, which can cause disease in the lungs, culture results must be interpreted in light of the patient's specific symptoms and overall condition.

The pathogenic organisms most often found in sputum include *Streptococcus pneumoniae*, *Mycobacterium tuberculosis*, *Klebsiella pneumoniae* (and other Enterobac-

Obtaining a specimen by nasotracheal suction

To collect a nasotracheal specimen, follow these steps.
• Gather the equipment you'll need: oxygen, 16 or 18 French suction catheter, water-soluble lubricant, sterile gloves, face mask, sterile in-line specimen trap, and normal saline solution.
• Attach the specimen trap to the suction catheter.
• Warn the patient that he'll experience some discomfort as the catheter passes into the trachea. If possible, place him in the high- or semi-Fowler position.
• Administer oxygen, as necessary.
• Because the patient may cough violently during suctioning, put on a mask to protect yourself from respiratory pathogens.
• After putting on sterile gloves, lubricate the catheter with normal saline solution.

• Ask the patient to hyperextend his head and extend his tongue.
• Pass the catheter through the patient's nostril. (Expect him to cough when the catheter passes through the larynx.)
• Advance the catheter into the trachea, and apply suction for no longer than 12 seconds. (If the patient becomes hypoxic or cyanotic, remove the catheter immediately and administer oxygen.)
• Stop the suction and gently remove the catheter.
• Administer oxygen, as necessary.
• Dispose of the catheter and gloves appropriately.
• Detach the in-line specimen trap from the suction apparatus. Cap the opening of the trap before you send it to the laboratory.

teriaceae), *Haemophilus influenzae*, *Staphylococcus aureus*, and *Pseudomonas aeruginosa*. Other agents, such as *Pneumocystis carinii*, *Legionella*, *Mycoplasma pneumoniae*, and respiratory viruses, may exist in the sputum and cause lung disease, but they usually require serologic or histologic diagnosis.

Stool culture

Bacteriologic examination of feces helps identify the pathogens causing GI disease. Such identification is vital not only to treat disease and prevent fatal complications, but also to confine the spread of severe infectious diseases—such as typhoid and dysentery.

If the stool culture doesn't show any unusual growth, nonbacterial gastroenteritis may be detected by immunoassay or electron microscopy.

Purpose
• To identify organisms causing GI disease
• To identify carrier states.

Procedure-related nursing care
Besides performing the nursing care discussed in the chapter introduction, take the following specific measures. Tell the patient how many stool specimens will be needed. (The test usually requires three specimens on consecutive days.) Explain that he'll need to avoid contaminating the specimen with toilet tissue or urine.

Instruct the patient to collect the

GI pathogens and associated conditions

The following list identifies pathogens that may appear in a stool culture, as well as several of the conditions they may cause.

☐ *Aeromonas hydrophila:* gastroenteritis, which causes diarrhea, especially in children
☐ *Bacillus cereus:* food poisoning, acute gastroenteritis (rare)
☐ *Campylobacter jejuni:* gastroenteritis
☐ *Clostridium botulinum:* food poisoning and infant botulism, a possible cause of sudden infant death syndrome
☐ *Clostridium difficile:* pseudomembranous enterocolitis
☐ *Clostridium perfringens:* food poisoning
☐ Enterotoxigenic *Escherichia coli:* gastroenteritis (resembles cholera or shigellosis)
☐ *Salmonella:* gastroenteritis, typhoid fever, nontyphoidal salmonellosis, paratyphoid fever
☐ *Shigella:* shigellosis, bacillary dysentery
☐ *Staphylococcus aureus:* food poisoning, enteritis or enterocolitis (when anti-infective therapy is used)
☐ *Vibrio cholerae:* cholera
☐ *Vibrio parahaemolyticus:* food poisoning, especially from seafood
☐ *Yersinia enterocolitica:* gastroenteritis, enterocolitis (resembles appendicitis), mesenteric adenitis, ileitis

stool specimen directly in the container. If he isn't ambulatory, you can collect the specimen in a clean, dry bedpan, then use a tongue blade to transfer the specimen to the container. Be sure you include any mucoid or bloody portions. And make sure the specimen represents the first, middle, and last portions of the feces passed.

If a rectal specimen is ordered, collect it with a sterile, rectal cotton-tipped swab. Insert the swab past the anal sphincter, rotate it gently, and withdraw it. Then place the swab in the appropriate container.

Place the specimen container in a leakproof bag before transporting it to the laboratory.

Normal results
About 96% to 99% of normal fecal flora consists of anaerobes, including non-spore-forming bacilli, clostridia, and anaerobic streptococci. The remaining 1% to 4% of normal fecal flora consists of aerobes, including gram-negative bacilli (predominantly *Escherichia coli* and other Enterobacteriaceae, plus small amounts of *Pseudomonas*), grampositive cocci (mostly enterococci), and a few yeasts.

Abnormal results
The most common pathogenic organisms of the GI tract are *Shigella, Salmonella,* and *Campylobacter jejuni.* (See *GI pathogens and associated conditions.*)

Throat culture

Used primarily to isolate and identify group A beta-hemolytic streptococci (such as *Streptococcus pyogenes*), a throat culture allows early diagnosis of pharyngitis and thus helps prevent sequelae, such as rheumatic heart disease and glomerulonephritis. The test can also screen for carriers of *Neisseria meningitidis.* Rarely, a throat culture is used to identify *Corynebacterium diphtheriae* or *Bordetella pertussis.*

Typically, the results of a throat culture are available in 2 to 3 days.

However, a fast-acting test can identify group A streptococci in only 7 minutes (see *Quick diagnosis of streptococcal pharyngitis*). Culture results must be evaluated in light of the patient's condition, his recent antibiotic therapy, and the number of normal flora.

Purpose

• To isolate and identify pathogens, particularly group A beta-hemolytic streptococci
• To screen asymptomatic carriers of pathogens, especially *N. meningitidis.*

Procedure-related nursing care

Besides performing the nursing care discussed in the chapter introduction, take the following specific measures. Explain to the patient that the collection procedure will take less than 30 seconds and that the results should be available in 2 to 3 days. Ask him about his immunization history if it's pertinent to the preliminary diagnosis. For example, was he immunized against pertussis?

Then tell the patient to tilt his head back and to open his mouth. Using a penlight and a tongue blade, check the throat for inflamed areas. With a cotton-tipped swab, wipe the tonsillar areas from side to side, touching any inflamed or purulent sites. Don't touch the patient's tongue, cheeks, or teeth with the swab.

Immediately place the swab in the culture tube. If you're using a commercial sterile collection and transport system, crush the ampule and force the swab into the medium to keep the swab moist until it gets to the laboratory.

Normal results

Normal throat flora includes nonhe-

Quick diagnosis of streptococcal pharyngitis

With a rapid, group A streptococcal test kit, you can identify group A streptococci in just 7 minutes. Using improved antibody-antigen technology, this test identifies the pathogens directly from the throat-culture swab.

The quick test results mean prompt diagnosis and treatment of streptococcal pharyngitis. However, this test doesn't identify any other pathogens that cause pharyngitis.

molytic and alpha-hemolytic streptococci, *Neisseria* species, some *Haemophilus* species, staphylococci, diphtheroids, pneumococci, yeasts, and enteric gram-negative rods.

Abnormal results

Possible pathogens include group A beta-hemolytic streptococci (*S. pyogenes*), which can cause scarlet fever or pharyngitis; *Candida albicans*, which can cause thrush; *Corynebacterium diphtheriae*, which can cause diphtheria; and *B. pertussis*, which can cause whooping cough.

Urine culture

Laboratory examination and culture of urine are used to evaluate urinary tract infections (UTIs) — most commonly bladder infections. Although urine in the kidneys and bladder is normally sterile, a small number of bacteria usually exist in the urethra. As a result, the urine specimen may contain various organisms. Despite this variety, however, bacteriuria usually results from a prevalence of a single type of

Centrifugation test

This test can quickly determine whether a patient's urinary tract infection originates in the upper urinary tract (kidneys) or the lower urinary tract (bladder). Here's how it works:

First, a urine specimen undergoes centrifugation. Then the sediment is stained with fluorescein. Viewed under a fluorescent microscope, the sediment fluoresces if the patient has an upper tract infection, but not if he has a lower tract infection.

bacterium. In fact, if the specimen contains more than two distinct bacterial species, it was probably contaminated during collection.

Because of the potential for contamination from the urethra and external genitalia, isolation of known pathogenic bacteria doesn't necessarily confirm UTI. Similarly, a single negative culture doesn't always rule out infection, as in chronic, low-grade pyelonephritis. Significant urine culture results are possible only after quantitative examination. To distinguish between bacteriuria and contamination, a clinician must know the number of organisms in a milliliter of urine—an estimate determined using a colony count. (For more information, see *Centrifugation test*.)

A clean-voided midstream collection is the method of choice for obtaining a specimen.

Purpose
● To diagnose UTI
● To monitor microorganism colonization after urinary catheter insertion.

Procedure-related nursing care
Besides performing the nursing care discussed in the chapter introduction, take the following specific measures.

Make sure your patient collects at least 3 ml of urine. The container, however, shouldn't be filled more than halfway. Wear clean gloves when you handle the specimen container. Send the specimen to the laboratory. If this can't be done within 30 minutes, store the specimen at 39.2° F (4° C) or place it on ice.

Normal results
Normal culture results are reported as "no growth"—a finding that usually indicates no UTI.

Abnormal results
Bacterial counts of 100,000 or more organisms of a single microbe species per milliliter of urine indicate probable UTI. Counts under 100,000/ml may be significant, depending on the patient's age, sex, history, and other factors. Counts under 10,000/ml usually suggest that the organisms are contaminants—except in symptomatic patients, those with urologic disorders, or those whose urine specimens were collected by suprapubic aspiration.

Pathogens may include *Escherichia coli, Proteus, Pseudomonas, Klebsiella, Aerobacter*, enterococci or, rarely, staphylococci.

Wound culture

Microscopic analysis of a wound culture can confirm infection in a lesion. Wound cultures may be aerobic (to detect organisms that usually require oxygen to grow and commonly appear in a superficial wound) or anaerobic (to detect organisms that need little or no oxygen and appear in areas of poor tissue perfusion, such as postoperative wounds, ulcers, or compound fractures). Indications for wound culture include fever, inflammation, and drainage from damaged tissue.

Purpose
• To identify an infectious microbe in a wound.

Procedure-related nursing care
Besides performing the nursing care discussed in the chapter introduction, take the following specific measures. Remove and discard any wound dressings. Wearing sterile gloves, prepare a sterile field and clean the area around the wound with antiseptic solution. (Never clean the area around a perineal wound.) The cleaning helps limit contamination of the culture by normal skin flora, such as diphtheroids, *Staphylococcus epidermidis*, and alpha-hemolytic streptococci. Make sure none of the antiseptic solution enters the wound.

Aerobic culture. To collect the specimen, express the wound and, using a sterile, cotton-tipped swab, collect as much exudate as possible. Or insert the swab deeply into the wound and gently rotate it. Place the swab in an aerobic culture tube immediately, and send it directly to the laboratory. Then dress the wound, as ordered.

Anaerobic culture. Collect the specimen for an anaerobic culture by inserting the sterile, cotton-tipped swab deeply into the wound. Place the swab in an anaerobic culture tube immediately because some anaerobes will die when exposed to even a small amount of oxygen.

Using an anaerobic specimen collector

Because some anaerobes die when exposed to the slightest bit of oxygen, tubes filled with carbon dioxide (CO_2) or nitrogen are used for oxygen-free transport.

The anaerobic specimen collector shown here consists of a rubber-stoppered tube filled with CO_2, a small inner tube, and a swab attached to a plastic plunger.

The tube on the left illustrates the position of the swab before you collect a specimen. You can see how the small inner tube containing the swab is held in place by the rubber stopper.

After collecting a specimen, you'll replace the swab in the inner tube and depress the plunger, as shown on the right. This action separates the inner tube from the stopper, forcing it into the larger tube — exposing the specimen to the CO_2-rich environment.

Before collection   **After collection**

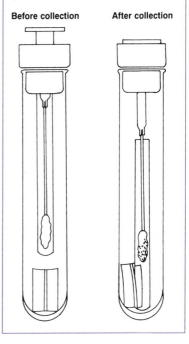

Make sure no air enters the tube and that the double stoppers on the tube are secure. (See *Using an anaerobic specimen collector,* page 85.)

You can also collect a specimen for an anaerobic culture by inserting a needle into the wound, aspirating 1 to 5 ml of exudate into a syringe, and immediately injecting the exudate into an anaerobic culture tube. If you're not using an anaerobic culture tube, you may cover the needle with a rubber stopper and send the aspirate to the laboratory in the syringe.

After collecting the specimen, dress the wound, as ordered.

Normal results
Pathogenic organisms normally aren't present in a clean wound.

Abnormal results
The most common aerobic pathogens in an infected wound include *Staphylococcus aureus*; group A beta-hemolytic streptococci; group D beta-hemolytic streptococci, including enterococci and *Streptococcus bovis*; Enterobacteriaceae; *Escherichia coli*; and some *Pseudomonas* species. The most common anaerobic pathogens include *Clostridium, Proteus*, and some *Bacteroides* species.

Suggested readings

Culla, J.H., and Watson, J. *Nurse's Manual of Laboratory Tests.* Philadelphia: F.A. Davis Co., 1989.

Diagnostics, 2nd ed. Nurse's Reference Library. Springhouse, Pa.: Springhouse Corp., 1987.

Fischbach, F.T. *A Manual of Laboratory Diagnostic Tests,* 3rd ed. Philadelphia: J.B. Lippincott Co., 1988.

Ravel, R. *Clinical Laboratory Medicine: Clinical Application of Laboratory Data,* 5th ed. Chicago: Year Book Medical Pubs., 1989.

Speicher, C.E. *The Right Test: A Physician's Guide to Laboratory Medicine.* Philadelphia: W.B. Saunders Co., 1989.

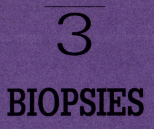

3

BIOPSIES

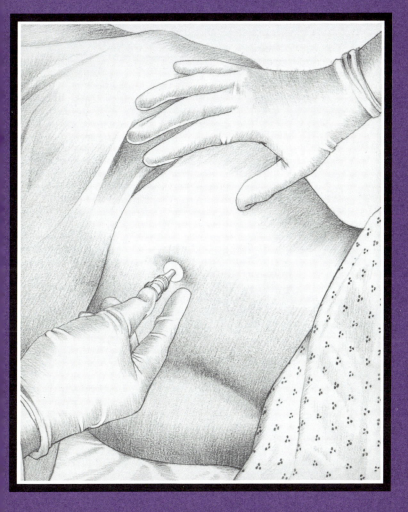

Vital to confirming cancer, biopsy involves extracting a small piece of living tissue from an organ or other body part for histologic examination. Over the years, biopsy techniques and needle designs have improved, allowing the removal of different types of specimens. For instance, a skilled practitioner can now rapidly remove a specimen from the deep tissues without surgery. (See *Understanding common tissue biopsies*.)

Biopsies commonly take place in a hospital but can also take place in a doctor's office or an outpatient surgical clinic. When the patient is hospitalized, the biopsy can be done at the bedside, in a treatment room, or in the operating room. Open biopsy, performed in the operating room, is typically necessary when results from closed biopsy or other tests (such as a computed tomography scan) suggest the need for complete excision of a tissue mass. Because complete excision of a tissue mass may be necessary, general anesthesia is commonly used.

Histologic examination

Depending on the situation, histologic examination is performed after standard tissue preparation, which can take several hours, or after frozen section, an alternate method of tissue preparation that permits pathologic diagnosis within 10 to 15 minutes after excision. The frozen section examination, although usually reliable, must be confirmed by standard preparation and analysis. In either case, an accurate histologic diagnosis by a pathologist depends on several factors:
● a representative or complete tissue specimen obtained using good technique to prevent tissue damage
● proper specimen handling, storage (usually in fixative), and preparation

● knowledge of the specimen's origin, the suspected diagnosis, any previous biopsies at the site, and any current treatments.

The pathologist's report after standard preparation and analysis will provide both gross and microscopic descriptions to aid histopathologic tissue classification of a tumor. A typical classification system involves a scale of four grades:
● G1 — well differentiated
● G2 — moderately well differentiated
● G3 — poorly differentiated
● G4 — anaplastic.

When the biopsy results confirm cancer, a staging system is used to direct treatment and make a prognosis. (See *TNM system of staging cancer*, page 90, for more information.)

Procedure-related nursing care

The following nursing care measures apply to all the biopsies discussed in this chapter. As part of the discussion of each biopsy, you'll also find specific nursing care considerations.

Before any procedure, tell the patient what to expect and answer any questions he has. Make sure the patient or a responsible family member has signed a consent form.

As necessary, help the patient assume the proper position for the procedure. If the patient is awake and alert, provide support throughout the procedure by talking quietly to him, describing what's being done and answering any questions.

After the procedure, apply an appropriate dressing to the biopsy site. Label the specimen appropriately and send it to the laboratory immediately. Monitor vital signs, as appropriate, and assess the biopsy site for excessive drainage. If the patient experiences pain at the site,

Understanding common tissue biopsies

BIOPSY TYPE AND TARGET TISSUE	EQUIPMENT	ADVANTAGES AND DISADVANTAGES
Excision Surgical removal of entire lesion from any tissue, possibly using local anesthetic	Scalpel	• *Advantage:* combines diagnosis and treatment of lesion • *Disadvantage:* may require major surgery with patient under general anesthesia
Shaving Tissue shaved from raised surface lesion on skin	Scalpel	• *Advantages:* generally safe; combines diagnosis and treatment of benign lesion; yields good cosmetic results • *Disadvantages:* may require excision or other treatment if lesion is malignant; may cause seeding of malignant cells
Needle Removal of core of tissue from bone, bone marrow, breast, lung, pleura, lymph node, liver, kidney, prostate, synovial membrane, or thyroid	Cutting needle (such as the Cope or Vim-Silverman cutting needle)	• *Advantages:* avoids need for surgery; usually furnishes a representative specimen; preserves cell architecture • *Disadvantages:* may require excision or other treatment based on histologic results; may be traumatic to surrounding tissues; may not furnish a representative specimen; may cause seeding of malignant cells
Aspiration Aspiration of tissue specimen from bone marrow or breast	Flexible or fine aspiration needle, needle guide, and aspiration syringe	• *Advantages:* avoids need for surgery; aspiration of fluid from a breast cyst combines diagnosis and treatment; fine-needle aspiration causes little pain and can be done for outpatients • *Disadvantages:* disturbs cell architecture; permits study of individual cells but not of intercellular structure; may not furnish a representative specimen; may cause seeding of malignant cells (less likely with fine-needle aspiration)
Punch incision Removal of tissue specimen from core of lesion in skin or cervix	Punch forceps	• *Advantages:* avoids need for surgery; furnishes a representative specimen • *Disadvantages:* may require excision or other treatment based on histologic results; may cause seeding of malignant cells when part of mass is removed

TNM system of staging cancer

The internationally recognized TNM staging system allows an accurate tumor description that can be adjusted as a patient's cancer progresses. This system helps in directing treatment and making prognoses. By ensuring reliable comparison of patients in various hospitals, the system also contributes to cancer research.

T for primary tumor
T refers to the anatomic extent of the primary tumor, based on its size, the depth of invasion, and the surface spread.
□ T_0: No evidence of primary tumor
□ T_1: A mobile, often superficial tumor (<2 cm in diameter) confined to the organ of origin
□ T_2: A localized tumor (2 to 5 cm in diameter) with some loss of mobility and deep extension into adjacent tissues
□ T_3: An advanced tumor (>5 cm in diameter) with complete loss of mobility, involving a region
□ T_4: A massive tumor (>10 cm in diameter) with extension into another organ (causing a fistula or sinus), major nerves, arteries and veins, or bone

N for nodal involvement
N addresses nodal size, mobility, and firmness; capsular invasion and the depth of invasion; the number of nodes involved; and ipsilateral, contralateral, bilateral, and distant node involvement.
□ N_0: No evidence of lymph node involvement
□ N_1: Palpable, mobile lymph nodes, limited to the first station; involved nodes are usually solitary, and larger (2 to 3 cm in diameter) and firmer than normal nodes
□ N_2: Palpable, partially mobile, firm to hard nodes (3 to 5 cm in diameter), limited to the first station; involved nodes may show capsular and partial matted muscle invasion, and contralateral or bilateral involvement
□ N_3: A node (>5 cm in diameter) with extension beyond the capsule and fixation to bone, large blood vessels, skin, or nerves
□ N_4: Fixed and destructive nodes (>10 cm in diameter) with extension to second or distant stations

administer analgesics as ordered. Also, be sure to provide emotional support to a patient awaiting diagnosis.

Bone marrow aspiration and biopsy

Bone marrow — the soft tissue contained in the medullary canals of long bone and in the interstices of cancellous bone — may be removed by aspiration or needle biopsy. Aspiration biopsy involves drawing a fluid specimen containing suspended marrow pustulae from the bone marrow. In needle biopsy, a core of marrow — cells, not fluid — is removed. These methods commonly are used concurrently to obtain the best possible marrow specimens.

Because bone marrow is the major site of hematopoiesis, histologic and hematologic examination of its contents provides reliable diagnostic information about blood disorders. Bone marrow biopsy is contraindicated in patients with severe bleed-

□ Nx: Nodes inaccessible to evaluation

M for metastasis

M refers to the presence or absence of metastasis.

□ M_0: No evidence of metastasis
□ M_1: Solitary metastasis
□ M_2: Multiple metastases in one organ with no or minimal functional impairment
□ M_3: Metastasis to multiple organs with no or minimal to moderate functional impairment
□ M_4: Metastasis to multiple organs with moderate to severe functional impairment
□ Mx: No metastatic workup done

Stages and survival rates

□ Stage I ($T_1 N_0 M_0$): 70% to 90% 5-year survival rate
□ Stage II ($T_2 N_1 M_0$): 50% to 70% 5-year survival rate
□ Stage III ($T_3 N_0 M_0$ or $T_{1-3} N_1 M_0$): 25% to 45% 5-year survival rate
□ Stage IV ($T_4 N_{0-1} M_0$; $T_{0-4} N_{2-3} M_0$; or $T_{0-4} N_{0-4} M_1$): 5% to 20% 5-year survival rate

ing disorders. Bleeding and infection may result from bone marrow biopsy at any site, but the most serious complications occur at the sternum. These rare complications include puncture of the heart and major vessels, causing severe hemorrhage, and puncture of the mediastinum, causing mediastinitis or pneumomediastinum.

Purpose

• To diagnose primary and metastatic tumors
• To diagnose thrombocytopenia, leukemias, granulomas, and aplastic, hypoplastic, and pernicious anemias
• To determine the cause of an infection
• To aid in staging a malignant disease, such as Hodgkin's disease
• To evaluate the effectiveness of chemotherapy and help monitor myelosuppression.

Procedure-related nursing care

Besides performing the nursing care discussed in the chapter introduction, take the following specific measures.

Before the procedure. Describe the procedure to the patient, explaining that it permits microscopic examination of a bone marrow specimen. Specify the selected biopsy site—the sternum, anterior or posterior iliac crest, vertebral spinous process, rib, or tibia. Explain that even though a local anesthetic will be administered, he'll probably feel some pressure during insertion of the needle and a brief, pulling pain on removal of the marrow.

Inform the patient that the doctor may require more than one bone marrow specimen. Also explain that a blood sample will be collected before the biopsy.

Check the patient's history for hypersensitivity to the anesthetic. As ordered, administer a mild sedative 1 hour before the procedure.

During the procedure. Position the patient so that the site can be exposed easily, and tell him to remain as still as possible during the procedure. Put on clean gloves so you can assist the doctor as necessary. Throughout the procedure, support the patient.

After the specimen is obtained, assist the doctor in preparing the marrow slides (if aspiration biopsy was performed) or in transferring

Bone marrow: Cell types and normal results

CELL TYPES	NORMAL RESULTS (MEAN)		
	Adults	Children	Infants
Normoblasts, total	25.6%	23.1%	8%
Pronormoblasts	0.2% to 1.3%	0.5%	0.1%
Basophilic	0.5% to 2.4%	1.7%	0.34%
Polychromatic	17.9% to 29.2%	18.2%	6.9%
Orthochromatic	0.4% to 4.6%	2.7%	0.54%
Neutrophils, total	56.5%	57.1%	32.4%
Myeloblasts	0.2% to 1.5%	1.2%	0.62%
Promyelocytes	2.1% to 4.1%	1.4%	0.76%
Myelocytes	8.2% to 15.7%	18.3%	2.5%
Metamyelocytes	9.6% to 24.6%	23.3%	11.3%
Bands	9.5% to 15.3%	0	14.1%
Segmented	6% to 12%	12.9%	3.6%
Eosinophils	3.1%	3.6%	2.6%
Basophils	0.01%	0.06%	0.07%
Lymphocytes	16.2%	16%	49%
Plasma cells	1.3%	0.4%	0.02%
Megakaryocytes	0.1%	0.1%	0.05%
Myeloid-erythroid ratio	2:3	2:9	4:4

the marrow into a labeled bottle containing Zenker's solution (if needle biopsy was performed).

Apply pressure for 5 minutes over the biopsy site to control the bleeding. Once the bleeding stops, clean the biopsy site, then apply either a sterile adhesive bandage or pressure dressing. If the doctor has performed an aspiration biopsy and a needle biopsy, you'll have to apply pressure to and dress two sites.

After the procedure. Monitor the patient's vital signs, and assess the dressing at the biopsy site or sites for excessive drainage. If the patient experiences pain at a biopsy site, administer an analgesic, as ordered.

For several days after the biopsy, monitor the patient for signs and symptoms of bone infection — fever, headache, pain on movement, and tissue redness or abscess at or near the biopsy site.

Normal results

Yellow marrow contains fat cells and connective tissue; red marrow contains hematopoietic cells, fat cells, and connective tissue. (See *Bone marrow: Cell types and normal results.*)

Stains that detect hematologic disorders normally produce these findings:
• iron stain, which measures hemosiderin (storage iron): +2 level
• Sudan black B (SBB) stain, which shows granulocytes: negative
• periodic acid-Schiff (PAS) stain, which detects glycogen reaction: negative.

Abnormal results

Histologic examination of a bone marrow specimen can help detect myelofibrosis, granulomas, lymphoma, or cancer.

Hematologic analysis, including the differential count and myeloid-erythroid ratio, can implicate a wide range of disorders. Elevated normoblast values are associated with polycythemia vera; depressed values, with vitamin B_{12} or folic acid deficiency and hypoplastic or aplastic anemia. Elevated neutrophil values suggest acute myeloblastic or chronic myeloid leukemia; depressed values, lymphoblastic or monocytic leukemia and aplastic anemia.

Elevated eosinophil levels occur in bone marrow carcinoma, lymphadenoma, myeloid leukemia, eosinophilic leukemia, and pernicious anemia (in relapse). Elevated lymphocyte levels are associated with chronic lymphocytic leukemia and other lymphoblastic leukemias, lymphomas, mononucleosis, aplastic anemia, and macroglobulinemia.

Elevated plasma cell levels are found in myelomas, collagen diseases, infection, antigen sensitivity, and cancer.

Elevated megakaryocyte values are associated with aging, chronic myeloid leukemia, polycythemia vera, megakaryocytic myelosis, infection, idiopathic thrombocytopenic purpura, and thrombocytopenia; depressed values, with pernicious anemia. An elevated myeloid-erythroid ratio is associated with myeloid leukemia, infection, leukemoid reactions, and depressed hematopoiesis; a depressed ratio, with agranulocytosis, hematopoiesis after hemorrhage or hemolysis, iron deficiency anemia, and polycythemia vera.

In an iron stain, decreased hemosiderin levels may indicate a true iron deficiency; increased levels may accompany other types of anemias or blood disorders. A positive SBB stain can differentiate acute granulocytic leukemia from acute lymphocytic leukemia (SBB-negative) or may indicate granulation in myeloblasts. A positive PAS stain may point to acute or chronic lymphocytic leukemia, amyloidosis, thalassemia, lymphomas, infectious mononucleosis, iron deficiency anemia, or sideroblastic anemia.

Nursing implications of abnormal results

If the test results confirm a hematologic cancer or another serious disorder, provide supportive care and good patient teaching to help the patient make the most of remissions and avoid or minimize complications.

Teach a patient with immunosuppression or neutropenia infection prevention measures, stressing the importance of promptly reporting any signs or symptoms of infection. Tell a patient with thrombocytopenia how to prevent bleeding. Emphasize the importance of detecting and reporting bleeding promptly.

Teach a patient with anemia the importance of getting adequate rest and eating a high-protein, iron-rich diet, if appropriate. Also be sure to provide instruction and support for any patient undergoing such treatments as chemotherapy or bone marrow transplant.

Breast biopsy

Although mammography, thermography, and X-rays aid in diagnosing breast masses, only a histologic examination of breast tissue obtained by biopsy can confirm or rule out cancer. Needle biopsy or fine-needle biopsy can provide a core of tissue or a fluid aspirate, but needle biopsy should be restricted to fluid-filled cysts and advanced malignant lesions. Both methods have limited diagnostic value because of the small and perhaps unrepresentative specimens they provide. Open biopsy provides a complete tissue specimen, which can be sectioned to allow more accurate evaluation. All three techniques require only a local anesthetic and commonly are performed on outpatients. However, if the patient is fearful or uncooperative, open biopsy may require a general anesthetic.

Breast biopsy is indicated for patients with palpable masses, suspicious areas revealed on a mammogram, bloody nipple discharge, or persistently encrusted, inflamed, or eczematoid breast lesions. Breast tissue analysis commonly includes an estrogen and progesterone receptor assay to help determine the most appropriate therapy if the mass proves malignant. This assay measures quick-frozen tumor tissue to determine the binding capacity of its estrogen and progesterone receptors.

Purpose
• To differentiate between benign and malignant breast tumors.

Procedure-related nursing care
Besides performing the nursing care discussed in the chapter introduction, take the following specific measures.

Before the procedure. Make sure you have a complete medical history. Be sure to ask when the patient first noticed the lesion, whether she feels any associated pain, and whether the size of the lesion has changed. Find out if a change in size is associated with the patient's menstrual cycle. Also ask about nipple discharge and any nipple or skin changes — such as the characteristic ''orange-peel'' skin that may indicate an underlying inflammatory carcinoma. Explain that pretest blood studies, urinalysis, and a chest X-ray may be required.

As you describe the procedure to the patient, explain that it allows microscopic examination of a breast tissue specimen. Offer emotional support, and reassure her that breast masses don't always indicate cancer. In fact, 80% of all breast lumps aren't malignant.

Check the patient's history for hypersensitivity to anesthetics. If she'll receive a general anesthetic, instruct her to fast from midnight the night before the procedure.

During the procedure. Assist the patient to either the sitting or recumbent position, as ordered. After the biopsy is completed, place the specimen in a properly labeled specimen bottle containing saline solution or formaldehyde (for needle biopsy), or formaldehyde only (for open biopsy). Apply pressure, then an adhesive bandage, to a needle biopsy site. After an open biopsy, the doctor will suture and dress the patient's wound.

After the procedure. If the patient received a local anesthetic, monitor her vital signs and provide medication for pain, as ordered. Watch for and report bleeding, tenderness, or redness at the biopsy site.

If the patient received a general anesthetic, check her vital signs every 15 minutes for 1 hour or until she's stable, then every 30 minutes for the next 4 hours, then every hour for the following 4 hours and, finally, every 4 hours thereafter for 24 hours. Continue to assess the site for bleeding, tenderness, and redness. If the patient complains of pain at the site, administer an analgesic, as ordered.

Normal results

Normally, breast tissue consists of cellular and noncellular connective tissue, fat lobules, and various lactiferous ducts. It appears pink and more fatty than fibrous, and shows no abnormal development of cells or tissue elements.

Abnormal results

Abnormal breast tissue may exhibit a wide range of benign or malignant pathologies. Benign tumors include fibrocystic disease, adenofibroma, intraductal papilloma, mammary fat necrosis, and plasma cell mastitis (mammary duct ectasia). Malignant tumors include adenocarcinoma, cystosarcoma, intraductal carcinoma, infiltrating carcinoma, inflammatory carcinoma, medullary or circum-

scribed carcinoma, colloid carcinoma, lobular carcinoma, sarcoma, and Paget's disease.

Nursing implications of abnormal results

If the biopsy confirms cancer, the patient will require emotional support to help her cope with the diagnosis, as well as an explanation and preparation for follow-up tests — including radiographic tests, blood studies, bone scans, and urinalysis — to determine the most appropriate treatment strategy.

Cervical punch biopsy

Indicated for women with suspicious cervical lesions, cervical punch biopsy consists of excising a tissue specimen for histologic examination, using sharp forceps. Performed when the cervix is least vascular (usually 1 week after menses), the procedure usually involves obtaining specimens from all areas with abnormal tissue or from the squamocolumnar junction and other sites around the cervical circumference. The selection of biopsy sites is based on cervical colposcopy (the most accurate method) or on Schiller's test, which stains normal squamous epithelium a dark mahogany but fails to color abnormal tissue. (Also see *Overview of endometrial and ovarian biopsies,* page 96.)

Purpose

• To evaluate suspicious cervical lesions
• To diagnose cervical cancer.

Procedure-related nursing care

Besides performing the nursing care discussed in the chapter introduc-

Overview of endometrial and ovarian biopsies

METHOD	PURPOSE	SPECIAL CONSIDERATIONS
Endometrial biopsy		
• Dilatation and curettage (D&C) • Endometrial washing (by jet irrigation, aspiration, or brushing)	• To evaluate uterine bleeding • To diagnose suspected endometrial carcinoma • To diagnose a missed abortion	• Time of menstrual cycle affects accuracy of biopsy results. • Type of specimen obtained depends on patient's age and disorder. • Endometrial washing requires no anesthesia and can be done in a doctor's office. • D&C may follow negative biopsy by endometrial washing. • Specimens obtained by D&C may be processed as frozen sections.
Ovarian biopsy		
• Transrectal or transvaginal fine-needle biopsy • Aspiration biopsy during laparoscopy	• To detect an ovarian tumor • To determine the spread of cancer	• Fine-needle biopsy may follow palpation, laparoscopy, or computed tomography that detects an abnormal ovary. • Aspiration during laparoscopy is particularly useful for young women who are infertile or who have lesions that appear benign.

tion, take the following specific measures.

Before the procedure. Describe the procedure to the patient, explaining that it provides a cervical tissue specimen for microscopic study. Tell her that she may experience mild discomfort during and after the procedure. Advise an outpatient to have someone accompany her home afterward. Just before the biopsy, have the patient void.

During the procedure. Place the patient in the lithotomy position. Encourage her to relax as the unlubricated speculum is inserted into the vagina.

After the biopsy is completed, help place each specimen in a labeled bottle containing 10% formaldehyde solution. To control bleeding, the doctor may swab the cervix with 5% silver nitrate solu-

tion. Or he may use cautery or sutures. If bleeding persists, a tampon may be inserted.

After the procedure. Instruct the patient to avoid strenuous exercise for 8 to 24 hours. Encourage an outpatient to rest briefly before leaving the office, short procedure unit, or clinic.

If a tampon was inserted after the biopsy, instruct the patient to leave it in place for 8 to 24 hours, as directed. Explain that some bleeding may occur, but tell her to promptly report bleeding that's heavier than her normal menses.

Emphasize the need to follow her doctor's instructions on tampon use because tampons can irritate the cervix and cause bleeding. Also reemphasize the doctor's instructions concerning douching and intercourse. These are usually restricted for 2 weeks or as directed.

Inform the patient that a foul-smelling, gray-green vaginal discharge is normal for several days after the biopsy and may persist for up to 3 weeks.

Normal results

Normal cervical tissue contains columnar and squamous epithelial cells, loose connective tissue, and smooth-muscle fibers, with no evidence of dysplasia or abnormal cell growth.

Abnormal results

Histologic examination of a cervical tissue specimen can identify abnormal cells and differentiate intraepithelial neoplasia from invasive cancer.

Nursing implications of abnormal results

If the cervical biopsy doesn't identify the cause of an abnormal Papanicolaou test, or if the specimen shows advanced dysplasia or carcinoma in situ, support the patient emotionally because she may be quite apprehensive. Anticipate a cone biopsy performed in the operating room with the patient under general anesthesia. A cone biopsy garners a larger tissue specimen, allowing more accurate evaluation.

Liver biopsy, percutaneous

Usually performed using a local anesthetic, this procedure involves needle aspiration of a liver tissue core for histologic analysis. Such analysis can identify hepatic disorders after ultrasonography, computed tomography, and radionuclide studies have failed to detect them.

Because many patients with hepatic disorders have clotting defects, testing for hemostasis should precede a liver biopsy. Percutaneous liver biopsy is contraindicated for a patient with a platelet count below 100,000/mm³; prothrombin time longer than 15 seconds; empyema of the lungs, pleurae, peritoneum, biliary tract, or liver; a vascular tumor; hepatic angiomas; a hydatid cyst; or tense ascites. If the doctor suspects an extrahepatic obstruction, he should order ultrasonography or subcutaneous transhepatic cholangiography to rule out the problem before performing a liver biopsy.

Purpose

• To diagnose hepatic parenchymal disease, cancer, and granulomatous infections.

Procedure-related nursing care

Besides performing the nursing care discussed in the chapter introduction, take the following specific measures.

Before the procedure. Describe the procedure to the patient, explaining that it helps diagnose liver disorders and answering any questions he has. Explain that he'll receive a local anesthetic but may experience pain similar to that of a punch in his right shoulder as the biopsy needle passes the phrenic nerve. Instruct him to restrict food and fluid intake for 4 to 8 hours before the procedure.

Check the patient's history for hypersensitivity to the local anesthetic. Ensure that prothrombin time and platelet count tests have been performed and that the results are recorded on the patient's chart. Just before the procedure, have the patient void.

Liver biopsy with a Menghini needle

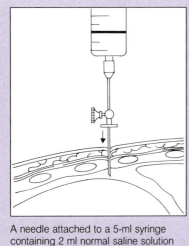

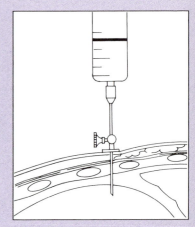

A needle attached to a 5-ml syringe containing 2 ml normal saline solution is introduced through the chest wall at the 8th or 9th right intercostal space. Approximately 1 ml of the solution is injected into the subcutaneous tissue.

The plunger is pulled back to create negative pressure. Then the needle is rapidly pushed into the liver.

During the procedure. For aspiration biopsy using a Menghini needle, assist the patient to the supine position with his right hand under his head. Tell him to maintain this position and to remain as still as possible during the procedure.

When the doctor is ready to insert the biopsy needle, he'll ask the patient to take a deep breath, then exhale and hold his breath to prevent chest wall movement. After the needle is withdrawn, instruct the patient to resume normal breathing. (See *Liver biopsy with a Menghini needle.*)

After the biopsy, assist the doctor in placing the tissue specimen in a properly labeled specimen cup containing 10% formalin solution. Apply pressure to the biopsy site to halt bleeding, then apply a dressing.

After the procedure. Position the patient on his right side for 2 hours, with a small pillow or sandbag under the costal margin to provide extra pressure. Advise the patient to remain in bed for 24 hours and to resume a normal diet as soon as he wishes.

After the procedure, assess the patient's vital signs every 15 minutes for the first hour or until he's stable, then every 30 minutes for the next 4 hours, then every hour for the next 4 hours and, finally, every 4 hours thereafter for 24 hours. Throughout this period, monitor him carefully for signs of shock.

Also watch for bleeding and for signs of bile peritonitis (tenderness and rigidity around the biopsy site). Be alert for signs and symptoms of pneumothorax, including an increas-

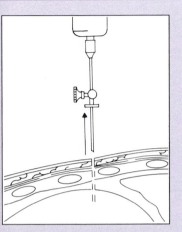

The needle is pulled out of the body entirely with the specimen in the syringe.

ing respiratory rate, diminished breath sounds, dyspnea, persistent shoulder pain, and pleuritic chest pain. If the patient complains of pain at the insertion site, administer an analgesic, as ordered.

Normal results
The normal liver consists of sheets of hepatocytes supported by a reticulin framework.

Abnormal results
Examination of hepatic tissue may reveal diffuse disease, such as cirrhosis or hepatitis, or granulomatous infections, such as tuberculosis. Primary malignant tumors include hepatocellular carcinoma, cholangiocellular carcinoma, and angiosarcoma; however, hepatic metastases are more common.

Nursing implications of abnormal results
If test results confirm a liver disorder, provide appropriate supportive care. Encourage the patient to recognize and cope with his illness. And try to promote independence and self-care.

You may also need to teach the patient how to prevent bleeding and detect it early. And you may instruct him on how to adjust his diet. Depending on his condition, you may need to monitor his neurologic status. If he has jaundice, take measures to ease his pain and discomfort. If he has ascites, tell him to remain calm and to try to breathe slowly.

Lung biopsy

Generally recommended after a chest X-ray, a computed tomography scan, and bronchoscopy have failed to identify the cause of diffuse parenchymal pulmonary disease or a pulmonary lesion, lung biopsy involves excising a pulmonary tissue specimen for histologic examination and microbiological analysis. Depending on the circumstances, a doctor may obtain the specimen using either closed or open technique. Closed technique includes both needle and transbronchial biopsies and requires only local anesthesia. Open technique, performed in the operating room with the patient under general anesthesia, involves both limited and standard thoracotomy.

Needle biopsy is appropriate for a readily accessible lesion or for a lesion originating in the lung parenchyma, confined to the parenchyma, or fixed to the chest wall. This tech-

Managing problems of lung biopsy

PROBLEM	SIGNS AND SYMPTOMS	NURSING INTERVENTIONS
Pneumothorax	• Sudden, sharp pleuritic pain • Dyspnea • Asymmetrical chest wall movements • Tachycardia • Anxiety, restlessness • Cyanosis	• Notify the doctor immediately. • Administer oxygen, monitor vital signs, and assess breath sounds. • Prepare to assist with needle aspiration of air and chest tube insertion.
Infection	• Warmth, redness, and swelling at biopsy site • Fever	• Notify the doctor. • Monitor vital signs.
Bleeding	• Hemoptysis after transbronchial biopsy • Blood-saturated dressing after needle biopsy	• Notify the doctor. • Monitor vital signs and assess breath sounds.

nique provides a much smaller specimen than that obtained with open technique. Needle biopsy is contraindicated for patients who have a lesion that's separated from the chest wall or accompanied by emphysematous bullae, cysts, or gross emphysema. The procedure is also contraindicated for those patients who have coagulopathy, hypoxia, pulmonary hypertension, or cardiac disease with cor pulmonale.

Transbronchial biopsy—removal of multiple tissue specimens through a fiber-optic bronchoscope—is appropriate when the patient has diffuse infiltrative pulmonary disease or tumors, or when severe debilitation contraindicates open biopsy.

Open biopsy generally is used to study a well-circumscribed lesion that may require resection.

Purpose
• To confirm a diagnosis of diffuse parenchymal pulmonary disease or pulmonary lesions.

Procedure-related nursing care
Besides performing the nursing care discussed in the chapter introduction, take the following specific measures.

Before the procedure. Describe the procedure to the patient, explaining that it helps diagnose lung tissue abnormalities. Tell him that a chest X-ray and blood studies (prothrombin time, activated partial thromboplastin time, and platelet count) will be done before the procedure and that another chest X-ray will be taken after the procedure. Instruct him to fast after midnight before the procedure. (If a local anesthetic will be used, the patient may be allowed to have clear liquids the morning of the test.)

Advise a patient who'll receive a local anesthetic that he may experience a sharp, transient pain when the biopsy needle touches the lung. Check the patient's history for hypersensitivity to the local anesthetic selected. As ordered, administer a mild sedative 30 minutes before the procedure to help the patient relax.

During the procedure. When assisting with a needle biopsy, have the patient sit upright with his arms folded on a table in front of him. Because coughing or movement can cause the biopsy needle to slip, possibly tearing the lung, instruct the patient to maintain this position throughout the procedure, to remain as still as possible, and to refrain from coughing. During the procedure, observe carefully for signs of respiratory distress — shortness of breath, tachycardia, and cyanosis.

After the doctor withdraws the biopsy needle, apply pressure to the biopsy site to stop the bleeding, then apply a small bandage.

After obtaining the tissue specimen, the doctor will divide it immediately. Help him place the tissue for histologic analysis into a properly labeled bottle containing 10% neutral buffered formaldehyde solution, and the tissue for microbiological analysis into a properly labeled sterile container. Send the specimens to the laboratory immediately.

After the procedure. Ensure that a repeat chest X-ray is done immediately after the biopsy is completed. Assess the patient's vital signs every 15 minutes for the first hour after the procedure, every 30 minutes for the next 4 hours, every hour for the following 4 hours, then every 4 hours for 24 hours. Watch for abnormal bleeding, dyspnea, tachycardia, diminished breath sounds on the biopsy side, and late-developing cyanosis. (See *Managing problems of lung biopsy.*)

Administer an analgesic, as ordered, to alleviate any discomfort.

Advise the patient to resume a normal diet as soon as he wishes.

Normal results
Normal pulmonary tissue shows uniform texture of the alveolar ducts, alveolar walls, bronchioles, and small vessels.

Abnormal results
Histologic examination of a pulmonary tissue specimen can reveal squamous cell or oat cell carcinoma, adenocarcinoma, or parenchymal pulmonary disease.

Nursing implications of abnormal results
Provide emotional support for the patient with a diagnosis of lung cancer. Encourage him to use the support and information resources available, such as the American Lung Association.

Suggested readings

Corbett, J.V. *Laboratory Tests and Diagnostic Procedures with Nursing Diagnoses,* 2nd ed. Norwalk, Conn.: Appleton & Lange, 1987.

Diagnostics, 2nd ed. Nurse's Reference Library. Springhouse, Pa.: Springhouse Corp., 1987.

Fischbach, F.T. *A Manual of Laboratory Diagnostic Tests,* 3rd ed. Philadelphia: J.B. Lippincott Co., 1988.

Kee, J.L. *Laboratory and Diagnostic Tests with Nursing Implications,* 3rd ed. Norwalk, Conn.: Appleton & Lange, 1990.

Ravel, R. *Clinical Laboratory Medicine: Clinical Application of Laboratory Data,* 5th ed. Chicago: Year Book Medical Pubs., 1989.

Speicher, C.E. *The Right Test: A Physician's Guide to Laboratory Medicine.* Philadelphia: W.B. Saunders Co., 1989.

4

RADIOGRAPHIC STUDIES

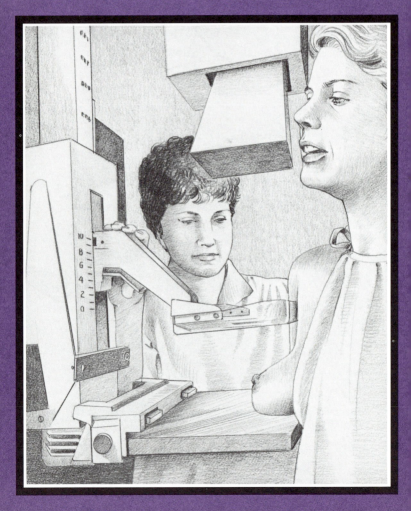

One of the most powerful diagnostic aids available, radiographic tests allow detailed study of both soft and bony tissues. These tests range from relatively simple studies, such as chest X-rays, to such complex studies as digital subtraction angiography. (See *Reviewing radiographic studies,* page 104.) Before focusing on commonly ordered tests, however, you should review some fundamentals—how the tests work, what risks they pose, and what your role will be.

How radiography works

Radiographic tests use X-rays, which are produced when high-voltage electrons strike a tungsten or molybdenum target in an X-ray tube. The tissues absorb, or attenuate, some of the radiation as it passes through the patient's body.

The radiation that isn't absorbed exposes the underlying X-ray film, producing an image in black, white, and shades of gray. The lighter areas on the film indicate denser tissue, such as bone. This tissue has already absorbed much of the radiation as it passed through the body, leaving less radiation to expose the film. Less-dense tissue, such as fat, lets more radiation pass through, producing the darker areas.

Risks of radiography

All radiographic studies pose certain risks. Two of the most common are radiation exposure and reactions to contrast media.

Radiation exposure. Radiation can harm not only the patient, but anyone else in or near the X-ray field. It may result in somatic effects that cause cellular damage and genetic effects that can harm future offspring.

Although all procedures pose some radiation risk, certain procedures pose a higher risk than others. For instance, fluoroscopy delivers a higher radiation dose than plain X-ray films. To keep doses within acceptable levels and lower the risks to the patient, federal and state agencies impose strict regulations on the radiation output per hour of fluoroscopy units.

To lower the radiation risk to staff members, personnel who don't have to be with the patient should leave the area during radiation exposure. Anyone who must remain should wear a protective lead apron and, if necessary, lead gloves. Lead-impregnated glasses can protect the operator's eyes during fluoroscopy.

Some patients—children, for example—are at greater risk from radiation. And, unless absolutely necessary, a pregnant patient shouldn't receive radiographic tests because of the risk to the fetus. When such tests are unavoidable, the patient's uterine region should be shielded with a lead apron.

Reactions to contrast media. Some procedures call for the use of a contrast medium to show details not visible on plain X-ray films. A contrast medium changes the radiopacity of one body part so it stands out against the surrounding area on the radiograph. But in some patients—especially those with a history of allergies—an iodinated contrast agent can cause life-threatening allergic or cytotoxic reactions. The risk increases when the contrast medium is injected intravenously or intra-arterially.

Anaphylaxis. A systemic hypersensitivity reaction to a sensitizing substance (such as a contrast medium), an anaphylactic reaction can range

Reviewing radiographic studies

TYPE AND DESCRIPTION	ADVANTAGES AND DISADVANTAGES
Plain films • Radiographs of bones and soft-tissue structures • Used for routine and general surveys	*Advantage* • Contrast agent not required *Disadvantage* • May not produce sufficiently detailed images
Fluoroscopy • Continuous X-ray imaging of body part • May use any type of contrast agent	*Advantage* • Provides dynamic imaging of body parts and contrast agents within them *Disadvantages* • Delivers higher radiation dose than plain films • May produce hypersensitivity reaction
Cineradiography • A motion-picture record of successive X-ray images • Uses I.V. contrast agent	*Advantage* • Allows dynamic imaging of structural and functional abnormalities *Disadvantages* • Delivers higher radiation dose than plain films • May produce hypersensitivity reaction
Tomography • Thin-section radiography that produces an image by moving the film and X-ray tube simultaneously in opposite directions to blur interfering structural shadows • Contrast agent used only during I.V. pyelography	*Advantage* • Permits clear view of thin sections of structures (bone tumors, for example) *Disadvantage* • Delivers higher radiation dose than plain films
Computed tomography • Cross-sectional axial tomography that, with computer assistance, produces a three-dimensional image • May use I.V. contrast agent to examine vasculature; may use diatrizoate meglumine (Gastrografin) or dilute barium to outline GI tract	*Advantage* • Allows detailed examination of soft tissues and bones *Disadvantage* • May produce hypersensitivity reaction
Angiography • Radiographic examination of blood vessels after introduction of intra-arterial or I.V. contrast agent	*Advantage* • Demonstrates tumors, infarcts, aneurysms, vascular injury, thromboses, stenoses, arteriovenous malformations, and arteriovenous fistulas *Disadvantage* • May produce hypersensitivity reaction
Digital subtraction angiography • Computer-assisted angiography that allows imaging of just the blood vessels containing intra-arterial or I.V. contrast agent	*Advantages* • Provides a clearer view of vessels than conventional angiography • Usually allows the use of less contrast agent than conventional angiography *Disadvantages* • Provides lower-resolution image with more artifacts than conventional angiography • May produce hypersensitivity reaction

from mild to severe. It can quickly become a medical emergency, leading to respiratory failure, hypovolemic shock, and death. You'll need to monitor the patient receiving a contrast agent carefully for signs of anaphylaxis, so he can receive immediate treatment if necessary. (See *Recognizing anaphylaxis.*)

Organ toxicity. The use of iodinated contrast agents can lead to nephrotoxicity, cardiotoxicity, and pulmonary toxicity.

Acute tubular necrosis or obstruction from contrast agent use can cause oliguria or anuria and possibly azotemia. The risk increases in patients with multiple myeloma, diabetic nephropathy, or preexisting renal failure. You can help prevent these reactions by making sure such patients receive enough fluids. A patient with poor renal function may also need hemodialysis or peritoneal dialysis to clear the contrast medium from the blood.

High doses or bolus injections of an iodinated contrast agent can produce such cardiotoxic effects as myocardial ischemia, cardiac arrhythmias, and conduction abnormalities. A patient with preexisting myocardial or valvular disease, atherosclerosis, or conduction disturbances runs the greatest risk of cardiotoxicity. Signs and symptoms of cardiotoxicity include chest pain, syncope, arrhythmias, and cardiac arrest.

Pulmonary toxicity may result in sludging of red blood cells in the pulmonary capillary bed. This in turn can increase pulmonary artery pressure—possibly leading to right ventricular failure—and decrease gas exchange at the alveolar level.

Procedure-related nursing care
The following nursing care mea-

COMPLICATIONS

Recognizing anaphylaxis

If your patient develops an anaphylactic reaction to a contrast medium, you may note some or all of the following:
- cutaneous effects—pruritus, erythema, urticaria, angioedema
- respiratory effects—lump in throat, hoarseness, coughing, sneezing, dyspnea, laryngeal edema, bronchospasms, stridor
- cardiovascular effects—hypotension, tachycardia, bradycardia, ischemia, myocardial depression
- GI effects—nausea, vomiting, diarrhea, abdominal cramps.

sures apply to all radiographic studies covered in this chapter. As part of the discussion of each study, you'll also find specific nursing care considerations.

Explain the test's purpose to the patient and describe the procedure, including the risks. He'll have concerns about these risks—especially the radiation dosage—so you need to give him accurate information to allay his fears and help him make an informed decision. Tell a pregnant woman that the doctor may postpone the test to protect the fetus.

Tell the patient where the procedure will take place. Usually, he'll go to the X-ray department, although testing sometimes takes place at the bedside.

Just before the procedure, make sure the patient removes all metal objects, such as jewelry or hairpins, that might block the X-rays.

Tell the patient he'll need to follow directions carefully to avoid repeating the test. For instance, he'll need to avoid moving while the

X-ray is taken to prevent blurring of the image.

Angiography

When radionuclide or computed tomography (CT) scanning suggests a vascular abnormality, a doctor may order an angiogram—a radiographic examination following injection of a radiopaque contrast medium into a vein or an artery.

To introduce the dye, the doctor will insert a catheter into the femoral or, less commonly, the brachial or carotid artery. He'll then use fluoroscopy to guide the catheter to the area to be visualized and inject the dye through the catheter. A series of rapid-sequence X-ray films is taken during injection and immediately afterward. These films show both the configuration and placement of the blood vessels. (For more information, see *Renal angiography.*)

Purpose
The purpose depends on the area being examined.

Cerebral angiography
● To detect cerebrovascular abnormalities, including aneurysm, arteriovenous malformation, thrombosis, and narrowing or occlusion
● To study vascular displacement caused by tumor, hematoma, edema, herniation, arterial spasm, increased intracranial pressure, or hydrocephalus
● To locate clips applied to blood vessels during surgery and to evaluate the postoperative status of such vessels.

Pulmonary angiography
● To detect pulmonary embolism in a symptomatic patient who has a normal or inconclusive lung scan
● To evaluate pulmonary circulation before surgery on a patient with congenital heart disease.

Renal angiography
● To demonstrate the configuration of the total renal vasculature before surgery and invasive procedures such as angioplasty
● To determine the cause of renovascular hypertension, including stenosis, thrombotic occlusions, emboli, and aneurysms
● To investigate renal masses and renal trauma
● To detect complications after renal transplantation, such as a nonfunctioning shunt or rejection of the donor organ.

Procedure-related nursing care
Besides performing the nursing care discussed in the chapter introduction, take the following specific measures.

Before the procedure. Tell the patient he'll be awake for the test. Explain the importance of remaining in the same position throughout the procedure, and warn him that holding this position may make his muscles feel stiff and sore for a short time afterward. Tell him he may feel transient nausea and a flushing and burning sensation during the injection of the contrast agent.

For pulmonary angiography, tell the patient that someone will monitor his heart rate throughout the procedure.

For renal angiography, check the doctor's orders and radiology procedure if the patient has compromised renal function. He may need acetazolamide before the procedure and I.V. solutions of mannitol and sodium bicarbonate before, during,

Renal angiography

Guided by fluoroscopy, the doctor advances a catheter up the femoroiliac vessels to the abdominal aorta and then into the renal artery. After he injects a contrast medium, the radiograph shows vessels during three phases of filling: arterial, nephrographic, and venous.

In a normal kidney, the contrast medium clearly defines the trunk and branches of the arterial tree during the arterial phase. During the nephrographic phase, the medium spreads from the renal arteries to the renal capillaries, concentrating in the pyramids and cortex. And during the venous phase, the contrast medium moves through the venous system.

Abnormal conditions may produce local retention of the contrast medium (indicating arterial stenosis), a bead-and-string filling pattern (a sign of arterial dysplasia), displacement or irregular branching of vessels, or unusual diffusion of the medium (indicating invasion by a tumor or cyst).

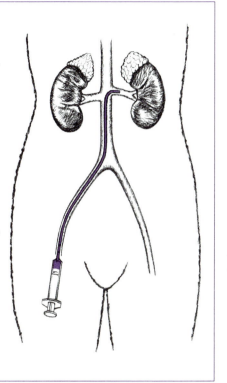

and after the procedure to prevent tubular obstruction. If so, explain this to the patient before the procedure.

Check the patient's history for hypersensitivity to iodine-based contrast media or iodine-containing foods, such as shellfish. If he has such a sensitivity, tell the doctor. He may prescribe a prophylactic antiallergenic, such as diphenhydramine or a steroid, or have one available during the procedure. Or he may cancel the test. Make sure the patient or a responsible family member has signed a consent form.

Tell the patient to fast for 8 hours before the procedure or as ordered.

Obtain baseline vital signs and, if ordered, administer a sedative or an analgesic 30 to 45 minutes before the test.

Have the patient void before he leaves his room.

During the procedure. If you're present for the procedure, give the following nursing care. Monitor the patient's vital signs throughout the procedure. For cerebral angiography, also monitor neurologic status.

After the doctor has injected the contrast agent, check for signs and symptoms of a hypersensitivity reaction, including dyspnea, nausea and vomiting, sweating, increased heart rate, and numbness in the extremities. Keep emergency resuscitation equipment nearby.

Once the X-rays have been taken and the catheter has been withdrawn, apply firm pressure to the puncture site for at least 15 minutes. Then cover the site with a pressure bandage. Check for bleeding and assess the distal pulses.

After the procedure. Make sure the patient rests in bed for 12 to 24 hours or as ordered. Give him pain medication, as ordered, and monitor his vital signs. If the patient had cerebral angiography, you'll also need to assess his neurologic status for 24 hours — every hour for the first 4 hours, then every 4 hours.

Monitor the patient's intake of I.V. fluids and his urine output. Unless contraindicated, make sure he receives extra fluids to help eliminate the contrast medium. Tell him he can resume his normal diet.

Look for bleeding or hematomas at the injection site. Keep the pressure dressing in place, and check the site every 30 minutes for 2 hours, then every hour for 4 hours. If you see bleeding, notify the doctor and apply direct pressure to the site. You can help ease discomfort and minimize swelling by applying an ice bag to the site.

Look for and report indications of a delayed hypersensitivity reaction to the contrast agent. These include dyspnea, pruritus, tachycardia, palpitations, hypotension or hypertension, excitation, and decreased urine output.

If the doctor injected the dye through the carotid artery, check for dysphagia or respiratory distress — signs of extravasation. Observe, too, for disorientation, and tell the patient to report weakness or numbness in the extremities — indications of thrombosis or hematoma. Also look for signs of transient ischemic attacks caused by arterial spasms. Report any of these signs or symptoms.

If the doctor used the brachial approach, immobilize the patient's arm for at least 12 hours and routinely check his radial pulse. Place a sign above his bed warning personnel not to take blood pressure readings in the affected arm. Monitor the arm and hand for any change in color, temperature, or tactile sensations — indicators of thrombosis or hematoma occluding the blood flow. If the arm becomes pale, cool, or numb, notify the doctor.

If the doctor used the femoral approach, keep the affected leg straight, usually for 8 to 12 hours or as hospital policy directs, and routinely check pulses distal to the site (dorsalis pedis and popliteal). Monitor the temperature, color, and tactile sensations in the leg to detect signs and symptoms of thrombosis, hematoma, or extravasation, which can stop blood flow.

Normal results
Blood vessels should have a normal structure and appear patent.

Abnormal results
Abnormal findings vary with the area examined.

Cerebral angiography. X-rays may confirm an aneurysm, arteriovenous malformation, thrombosis, stenosis, or occlusion, or they may show vascular changes caused by a tumor, hematoma, cyst, edema, herniation, arterial spasm, or hydrocephalus.

Pulmonary angiography. X-rays may show an interrupted blood flow resulting from pulmonary emboli, vascular filling defects, or stenosis.

Renal angiography. Hypervascularity on X-rays may signal renal tumors. A noticeable constriction in the blood vessels indicates renal artery stenosis. Alternating aneurysms and stenotic regions result from renal artery dysplasia, and reduced vascularity may stem from severe or chronic pyelonephritis. X-rays also may show other renal disorders, including infarction, arterial aneurysm, arteriovenous fistula, tissue distortion and fibrosis, abscess, cyst, intrarenal hematoma, parenchymal laceration, and fractured kidney.

Nursing implications of abnormal results
If angiography confirms the need for medical treatment, follow the recommended treatment plan.

Barium enema

A barium enema consists of a radiographic study of the large intestines after rectal instillation of barium sulfate (a radiopaque contrast medium) and, usually, air. This test is indicated for patients who have a history of altered bowel habits, lower abdominal pain, unexplained weight loss, or blood, mucus, or pus in the stool.

Guided by fluoroscopy, the doctor introduces the barium through a rectal tube into the large intestine. To help the barium fill the intestine, the doctor tilts the X-ray table or places the patient in the supine, prone, or lateral decubitus position. The procedure rarely causes complications, although it can result in a perforated colon or water intoxication.

Although a barium enema clearly outlines most of the large intestine, proctosigmoidoscopy provides the best view of the rectosigmoid region. A barium enema should precede a barium swallow and an upper GI and small-bowel series because ingested barium may take several days to pass through the GI tract, interfering with subsequent X-ray studies.

Purpose
● To help diagnose inflammatory disease
● To detect lesions, polyps, diverticula, and structural changes in the large intestine.

Procedure-related nursing care
Besides performing the nursing care discussed in the chapter introduction, take the following specific measures.

Before the procedure. Tell the patient the test will take roughly 1½ to 2 hours. Warn him that he'll feel full during the procedure and will experience moderate to severe cramping, the urge to defecate, and generalized abdominal discomfort as the barium and air enter the intestine. Reassure him that these sensations will pass quickly. Make sure the patient understands that accurate test results depend on his following dietary restrictions and bowel preparation. (See *Preparing for a barium enema,* page 110.)

During the procedure. If you're present for the procedure, give the following nursing care. Instruct the patient to breathe deeply and slowly through his mouth to ease discomfort as the barium and air enter the intestine. Tell him to keep his anal

Preparing for a barium enema

To prepare for a barium enema the following morning, your patient will need to follow these dietary and medication guidelines.

Day before the test
☐ *12 noon:* For lunch, follow a clear liquid diet without milk.
☐ *1 p.m.:* Drink an 8-oz glass of water.
☐ *3 p.m.:* Drink an 8-oz glass of water.
☐ *5 p.m.:* For supper, follow a clear liquid diet without milk.
☐ *7 p.m.:* Drink a full bottle of cold magnesium citrate.
☐ *9 p.m.:* Swallow three bisacodyl (Dulcolax) tablets whole with a glass of water.

Day of the test
☐ *12 midnight:* Stop taking all food and drink.
☐ *6 a.m.:* Insert a bisacodyl suppository rectally and drink 12 oz of water.

sphincter tightly contracted against the rectal tube to hold it in position and help keep the barium from leaking.

After the procedure. Before letting the patient have any food or fluids, make sure the doctor hasn't ordered any further X-rays. If he hasn't, encourage the patient to drink extra fluids, as ordered, to compensate for any dehydration the bowel preparation and the test may have caused. Also make sure he rests as much as possible because the bowel preparation and the procedure itself exhaust most patients.

As ordered, administer a mild cathartic or cleansing enema to counteract possible intestinal obstruction or fecal impaction from barium retention. Tell the patient his stool

will be lightly colored for 24 to 72 hours. Record a description of any stool passed by the patient in the hospital.

Normal results
Barium should fill the colon uniformly and reveal a normal contour, patency, position, and mucosal pattern on X-rays.

Abnormal results
A barium enema may reveal carcinoma, diverticulitis, chronic ulcerative colitis, granulomatous colitis, polyps, intussusception, gastroenteritis, stenosis, irritable colon, Hirschsprung's disease, and some cases of acute appendicitis.

Nursing implications of abnormal results
If the test results indicate a colon disorder, prepare the patient for further tests as ordered. For instance, if the test results suggest colon cancer, he'll need a biopsy. As necessary, explain the recommended medical regimen or surgical intervention to the patient.

Cholangiography, postoperative

Performed 7 to 10 days after cholecystectomy or common bile duct exploration, postoperative (or T-tube) cholangiography allows further examination of the biliary ducts. In this procedure, a contrast medium, injected through a T tube, flows through the biliary ducts and outlines the size and patency of the ducts. (The T tube is already in place to promote drainage from earlier surgery.) Radiographic and fluo-

Operative cholangiography

An alternative to postoperative cholangiography, operative cholangiography helps confirm a diagnosis in cases of suspected cholelithiasis or jaundice resulting from calculi in the biliary tree. In this test, the doctor injects a contrast medium, such as diatrizoate sodium, through a thin needle or catheter directly into the common bile duct, the cystic duct, or the gallbladder during surgery. If the gallbladder has been removed before injection, the doctor can insert a T tube, as shown below, and deliver the contrast medium through it (operative T-tube cholangiography).

As the contrast medium flows through the biliary ducts, it may reveal calculi and small intraluminal neoplasms, permitting the doctor to remove them before closing the incision. Although operative cholangiography can eliminate the need for further surgery, this advantage must be weighed against the risks associated with administering a contrast medium during a simple cholecystectomy.

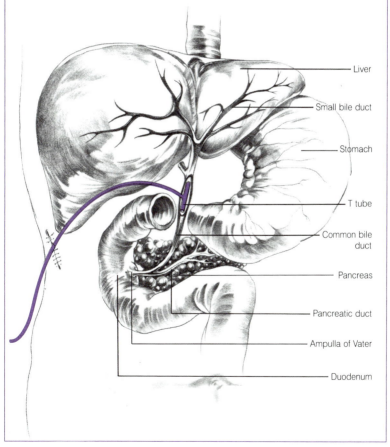

Liver

Small bile duct

Stomach

T tube

Common bile duct

Pancreas

Pancreatic duct

Ampulla of Vater

Duodenum

roscopic examination can then reveal any obstruction overlooked during surgery. (Also see *Operative cholangiography,* page 111.)

Purpose
• To detect strictures, calculi, neoplasms, and fistulas in the biliary ducts.

Procedure-related nursing care
Besides delivering the nursing care discussed in the chapter introduction, perform the following specific measures.

Before the procedure. Warn the patient that he may feel a sensation of pressure and epigastric fullness as well as transient back pain in his upper right side during the injection of the contrast medium. Reassure him that these sensations will pass.

Check his history for hypersensitivity to iodine-based contrast media or iodine-containing foods, such as shellfish. If he has such a sensitivity, tell the doctor. He may prescribe a prophylactic antiallergenic or cancel the test. Also make sure the patient or a responsible family member has signed a consent form.

Clamp the T tube the day before the procedure, as ordered. This causes bile to fill the tube, helping prevent air bubbles from entering the ducts. (On the radiograph, such air bubbles may resemble calculi.)

During and after the procedure. If you're present for the procedure, monitor the patient for indications of a hypersensitivity reaction. After the procedure, monitor the patient's vital signs. Report indications of a delayed hypersensitivity reaction to the contrast medium. Unless contraindicated, make sure the patient receives extra fluids to help him eliminate the medium.

If the doctor has removed the T tube, check the site periodically. Note any drainage, and change the sterile dressing as necessary. If the doctor has left the T tube in place, attach it to the drainage system, as ordered.

Normal results
Biliary ducts normally appear patent, with no strictures, calculi, neoplasms, or fistulas.

Abnormal results
The cholangiogram may uncover strictures, calculi, neoplasms, or fistulas overlooked during surgery.

Nursing implications of abnormal results
If the results indicate retained calculi, expect that the T tube will remain in place—usually for about 3 weeks—until it establishes a tract. Explain to the patient that the doctor will try to remove the calculi nonsurgically by removing the T tube and inserting a basket catheter through the T-tube tract into the common bile duct.

Cholecystography

A painless and noninvasive test, oral cholecystography allows radiographic examination of the gallbladder after the patient ingests a contrast medium. Most commonly used to confirm gallbladder disease, cholecystography is also indicated for patients with signs and symptoms of biliary tract disease, such as upper right quadrant pain, fat intolerance, and jaundice.

After ingestion, the contrast medium is absorbed by the small intestine, filtered by the liver, excreted into the bile, and then concentrated and stored in the gallbladder. In 12 to 14 hours, the gallbladder usually becomes opaque, and a series of X-ray films then records its appearance. If the patient also takes a fat stimulus, the gallbladder will contract and empty the bile into the common bile duct and small intestine. X-rays then allow the doctor to evaluate this process.

A gallbladder that fails to opacify or becomes only faintly opaque may signal an inflammatory disease, such as cholecystitis, with or without gallstones. The inflammation impairs the ability of the gallbladder mucosa to concentrate the contrast medium, preventing or diminishing opacification. Gallstones may add to the problem by obstructing the cystic duct, preventing contrast medium from entering the gallbladder.

A gallbladder that doesn't contract after the patient eats a fatty meal may signal cholecystitis or common bile duct obstruction. If the X-ray films don't pinpoint the cause, the patient may need to repeat the procedure the next day.

Purpose
• To detect gallstones
• To help diagnose inflammatory disease and gallbladder tumors.

Procedure-related nursing care
Besides performing the nursing care discussed in the chapter introduction, take the following specific measures.

Before the procedure. Tell the patient he'll have X-rays taken 12 to 14 hours after he ingests an oral contrast agent. Explain that he'll need to assume various positions on the radiographic table during the procedure.

Check the patient's history for hypersensitivity to contrast media. If he has such a sensitivity, tell the doctor, who may order a prophylactic antiallergenic or cancel the test. Make sure you schedule the test before any barium study.

If ordered, give the patient a meal containing fat at noon the day before the test and a fat-free meal that evening. The fat in the first meal stimulates the gallbladder to release bile. The second meal inhibits gallbladder contraction, causing the bile to accumulate.

After the evening meal, restrict all food and fluids except water. As ordered, give the patient six tablets of iopanoic acid 2 to 3 hours after the evening meal. (The doctor may order another contrast agent, such as ipodate, but iopanoic acid is used most frequently.) Have the patient swallow the tablets one at a time at 5-minute intervals, with one or two mouthfuls of water. He should drink a total of 8 oz of water with the tablets and drink nothing more until after the test. Warn him that the iopanoic acid commonly causes diarrhea and sometimes results in nausea and vomiting, abdominal cramps, and painful urination. He should tell you at once if any of these signs or symptoms develops.

Examine any vomitus or diarrhea for undigested tablets. If you find any, tell the doctor and the X-ray department personnel.

During and after the procedure. If you're present for the procedure, monitor the patient for signs and symptoms of a hypersensitivity reaction. After the procedure, make sure the patient drinks extra fluids to help eliminate the medium, unless contraindicated.

If the doctor orders the test repeated, keep the patient on a low-fat diet until the next test.

Normal results
On the X-rays, the gallbladder should look normal in size and structure with no evidence of inflammation or gallstones.

Abnormal results
An abnormal cholecystogram may point to gallstones (cholelithiasis), cholecystitis, cholesterol polyps, or a tumor, such as adenomyoma.

Nursing implications of abnormal results
If the X-rays reveal small gallstones, teach the patient to follow a fat-restricted diet to help prevent recurrent attacks. If the X-rays reveal large gallstones or a disease that requires surgery, find out what type of surgery is needed. Explain the procedure to the patient, answer any questions, and prepare him for surgery, as indicated.

Computed tomography

Computed tomography (CT) provides a three-dimensional image of a portion of the body. It does this by passing multiple X-ray beams from a computerized scanner (a hundred times more sensitive than an X-ray machine) through the body at different angles, creating a series of cross-sectional views, or anatomic slices. A computer then reconstructs these views into a three-dimensional image on a video screen and keeps a permanent record of that image.

The variations in brightness in the three-dimensional image — ranging from black through gray to white — reflect the amount of radiation absorbed by different areas in the tissue. The more dense the tissue, the more radiation it absorbs,

and the lighter it appears on the CT image. Thus, the test is especially useful for detecting the differences in tissue density caused by tumors. With small tumors, a radiopaque contrast medium can help enhance the image.

CT scans can provide images of almost any body area, including the head, orbit of the eye, thorax, spine, biliary tract and liver, kidneys, and pancreas. (See *How a CT scanner works.*)

Purpose
• To detect and evaluate tumors and other abnormalities
• To differentiate calcifications and cysts from tumors
• To monitor the effects of surgery, radiation therapy, or chemotherapy on tumors.

Procedure-related nursing care
Besides performing the nursing care discussed in the chapter introduction, take the following specific measures.

Before the procedure. Tell the patient he'll lie on an X-ray table with his head or body (depending on the area being scanned) inside a scanning tunnel. Explain that the scanner will make loud, clacking sounds as it rotates around him but that the scan is painless. Emphasize that he must lie still when asked, or his movements may distort the images. Tell him the test takes about 15 minutes to an hour and a half.

If the doctor orders an I.V. contrast medium, tell the patient he may feel brief discomfort from the needle puncture and a localized sensation of warmth during the injection. Warn him that he may also develop a passing headache, feel nauseated, or notice a salty or metallic taste, but that these reactions will last for only about a minute.

For a scan of the biliary tract and liver or the pancreas, or any scan that calls for a contrast medium, instruct the patient to fast — after midnight the night before the test for a morning scan or for 4 hours before an afternoon test. He doesn't need to fast for a renal, intracranial, spinal, thoracic, or orbital CT scan without a contrast medium.

If the doctor plans to use a contrast medium, check the patient's history for hypersensitivity reactions. Report any such reactions to the doctor, who may order a prophylactic medication or choose not to use contrast enhancement. Have the patient or a responsible family member sign a consent form.

If the patient seems apprehensive, tell the doctor and, if ordered, administer a sedative. Just before a biliary tract and liver scan or a pancreatic scan, administer an oral contrast medium, if ordered.

During and after the procedure. If you're present for the procedure, encourage the patient to relax and lie quietly. If he has received a contrast medium, monitor him for an allergic reaction.

After the procedure, monitor the patient who received a contrast medium for residual adverse reactions, including headache, nausea, and vomiting. Unless contraindicated, provide extra fluids to help him eliminate the dye. Tell him he can resume his normal diet.

Normal results

The structure scanned should have a normal size, shape, position, and density.

Abnormal results

A CT image that shows areas of altered density, a displaced structure,

How a CT scanner works

A computed tomography (CT) scanner allows detailed study of a portion of the body by creating a three-dimensional image. In intracranial CT, for example, the CT scanner encircles the patient's head. An X-ray tube inside the scanner emits multiple X-ray beams as the scanner rotates around the patient's head (see arrows). These X-ray beams pass through the patient's head and are picked up by detectors. A computer then translates the X-rays into a three-dimensional image on a video screen. The image clearly defines intracranial structures — an improvement over conventional X-rays, which blur the structures into black and white masses.

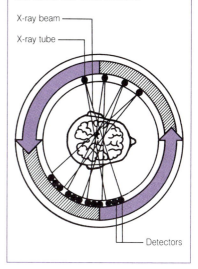

or a structure with an altered size or shape indicates a disorder.

Intracranial CT. An abnormal image may indicate intracranial tumors, cysts, or calcifications; cerebral atrophy, infarction, or edema; brain abscess; hydrocephalus; arteriovenous malformation; or epidural, subdural, or intracerebral hematomas.

Orbital CT. A CT scan of the eye's orbit may show an infiltrative lesion, but it can't identify the type of lesion. It also can help pinpoint the cause of unilateral exophthalmos (for example, lesions in the ethmoid sinus or in the orbital or paranasal sinuses), identify thickening of the medial and lateral rectus muscles resulting from Graves' disease, and confirm the presence of hemorrhage or tumor in the optic nerve sheath.

Thoracic CT. The scan may indicate tumors, nodules, cysts, aortic aneurysms, enlarged lymph nodes, pleural effusion, parenchymal diseases such as pneumonia, or the accumulation of blood, fluid, or fat.

Spinal CT. The CT image may show a spinal lesion or abnormality, such as a tumor or paraspinal cyst. It also reveals degenerative processes and structural changes, such as cervical spondylosis, herniated nucleus pulposus, and congenital spinal malformations such as meningocele.

Biliary tract and liver CT. The scan may indicate primary or metastatic hepatic neoplasms; hepatic abscesses, cysts, or hematomas; or dilated biliary ducts, a sign of obstructive rather than nonobstructive jaundice. The scan can also show the cause of biliary obstruction — calculi, for instance.

Renal CT. An abnormal scan may result from renal cysts, tumors, or calculi; adrenal tumors; polycystic kidney disease; congenital anomalies of the kidneys; perirenal hematomas; lymphoceles; or abscesses.

Pancreatic CT. The CT image may point to acute or chronic pancreatitis, pancreatic carcinoma, benign pancreatic tumor, or pancreatic abscesses or pseudocysts.

Nursing implications of abnormal results
If the test results indicate a disorder, give the patient and his family emotional support and follow the recommended treatment plan.

Digital subtraction angiography

A sophisticated radiographic technique, digital subtraction angiography (DSA) uses video equipment and computer-assisted image enhancement to examine the vascular system. DSA is useful in detecting lesions missed by computed tomography scans, such as thromboses of the superior sagittal sinus.

As in conventional angiography, X-ray images are taken after injection of a contrast medium. But unlike conventional angiography, in which images of bone and soft tissue commonly obscure vascular detail, DSA provides a high-contrast view of blood vessels without interfering images or shadows.

Digital subtraction makes this unique view possible. Here's how: A computer converts fluoroscopic images taken before and after injection of a contrast medium into digital information. The computer then "subtracts" the first image from the second, eliminating most information (mainly bone and soft tissue) common to both images. This results in a clearer image of the contrast agent-enhanced vasculature.

DSA usually calls for I.V. injection of the contrast medium, not intra-arterial injection, the most common method used in conventional angiography. To evaluate vascular anatomy, however, an intra-arterial injection may be necessary. The I.V. injection avoids one risk of conventional angiography — stroke — as well as the pain of arterial catheterization. The most common I.V. injection sites are the antecubital basilic and cephalic veins.

Purpose

• To visualize extracranial and intracranial cerebral blood flow
• To diagnose arteriovenous malformations, aneurysms, and vascular tumors
• To detect and evaluate cerebrovascular abnormalities, such as carotid stenosis and occlusion
• To visualize displacement of vasculature by other intracranial disorders or trauma
• To aid postoperative evaluation of cerebrovascular surgery, such as arterial grafts and endarterectomies.

Procedure-related nursing care

Besides performing the nursing care discussed in the chapter introduction, take the following specific measures.

Before the procedure. Tell the patient he'll probably feel some brief discomfort from the insertion of a needle or catheter used to introduce the contrast medium. The medium may also cause a feeling of warmth, a headache, a metallic taste, and nausea and vomiting. Reassure him that these sensations will pass quickly.

Check the patient's history for hypersensitivity reactions to radiographic contrast media. Report any such reactions to the doctor, who may order a prophylactic medication or cancel the test. Make sure the patient or a responsible family member has signed a consent form.

Tell the patient that he'll need to fast for 4 hours before the test but that he can have fluids.

During the procedure. If you're present for the procedure, monitor the patient's vital signs. For a cerebral DSA, also monitor his neurologic status. Observe the patient for indications of a hypersensitivity reaction, including urticaria, flushing, and respiratory distress.

After the procedure. Periodically check the venipuncture site for redness, swelling, and bleeding. If a hematoma develops, elevate the arm and apply warm soaks; if bleeding develops, apply firm pressure to the puncture site.

Because the contrast medium acts as a diuretic, encourage the patient to drink extra fluids over the next 24 hours. Tell him the fluids will also help him quickly excrete the contrast medium. Monitor his fluid intake and output, as ordered.

Monitor the patient for a delayed hypersensitivity reaction. Although rare, such reactions can occur up to 18 hours after the procedure.

Tell the patient he can resume his normal diet.

Normal results

The study should reveal normal vasculature.

Abnormal results

DSA may reveal aneurysms, arteriovenous occlusion, or stenosis, possibly from vasospasm. The test may also indicate vascular malformation or angiomas, arteriosclerosis, and cerebral embolism or thrombosis. The image may show vessel displacement or vascular masses (signs of an intracranial tumor) as well as the vascular supply of some tumors.

Nursing implications of abnormal results

If the test reveals a disorder, prepare the patient physically and emotionally for further treatment, such as vascular or tumor surgery.

Mammography

Mammography highlights differences in the density of breast tissue to help detect and evaluate cysts and tumors, especially those that aren't palpable. Mammography can detect between 90% and 95% of all breast cancers. A biopsy of suspicious areas confirms a diagnosis.

In this procedure, the patient rests her breast on a table above an X-ray cassette. Then the compressor, placed on the breast, takes an X-ray. The machine rotates and takes another X-ray from a different angle. The procedure is repeated on the other breast.

A variation of mammography, xeromammography uses less radiation, provides a higher-contrast picture, and gives more accurate results than regular mammography. In this procedure, a selenium-coated plate under the breast photoelectrically records the xerogram on paper.

The American Cancer Society, the American College of Radiology, and the American College of Obstetricians and Gynecologists provide guidelines for women to follow in obtaining mammograms (see *Guidelines for mammography*).

A woman shouldn't undergo mammography during pregnancy because her breasts become engorged and more sensitive. Also, despite shielding of the abdomen, internal radiation scattering can still occur. A biopsy takes the place of a mammogram during pregnancy if a woman has suspicious lumps.

Purpose

- To screen for breast cancer
- To investigate palpable and unpalpable breast masses, breast pain, or nipple discharge
- To help differentiate benign breast disease from breast cancer.

Procedure-related nursing care

Besides performing the nursing care discussed in the chapter introduction, take the following specific measures. Before the procedure, ask the patient if she's pregnant and document her response. If she knows or suspects that she's pregnant, tell the doctor. If she suspects she's pregnant, schedule a pregnancy test. After a negative pregnancy test, you can reschedule the patient for the mammogram.

Tell the patient the procedure takes about 15 minutes. Instruct her not to use powder, ointment, or deodorant on her breasts or under her arms the day of the test.

CHECKLIST

Guidelines for mammography

Use this checklist to advise patients on when they should obtain mammograms.

☐ A woman between ages 35 and 40 should obtain a baseline mammogram.

☐ A woman between ages 40 and 49 should have a mammogram every 1 or 2 years, based on the initial mammogram and other risk factors.

☐ A woman age 50 and older should have a mammogram once a year.

Just before the test, give the patient a gown to wear that opens in the front. If you're present for the procedure, provide emotional support. The patient may find that having her breast compressed during the X-ray is uncomfortable.

After the procedure, answer her questions and tell her how she can find out the test results.

Normal results
A mammogram should reveal normal mammary ducts, glandular tissue, and fat distribution. No abnormal masses or calcifications should appear.

Abnormal results
Well-outlined, regular, and clear spots suggest benign cysts. Irregular, branching, poorly outlined, opaque areas suggest a malignant tumor. Benign cysts tend to occur bilaterally; malignant tumors are usually solitary and unilateral.

Nursing implications of abnormal results
If the mammogram suggests an abnormality, provide emotional support. Assess the patient's level of understanding, and encourage her to tell you her concerns. Answer any questions she may have.

As ordered, prepare her for other studies, such as ultrasonography, computed tomography, magnetic resonance imaging, and diaphanography. She may also need an aspiration study or a needle biopsy.

Plain X-rays

Used for routine and general survey purposes, plain X-rays produce two-dimensional images of bones and soft-tissue structures without using any contrast agents. These plain X-rays allow a doctor to examine several areas and structures of the body, including the head and neck; the chest; the kidneys, ureters, and bladder; the abdomen; and the skeleton.

Usually, plain X-rays are performed in the radiology department. However, in certain circumstances, a portable X-ray may be done at the patient's bedside (see *Assisting with a portable chest X-ray,* page 120).

Purpose
The purpose varies with the area examined.

Head and neck
● To detect fractures from head trauma
● To help detect and assess tumors, calcifications, infections, bleeding, and increased intracranial pressure (ICP)
● To look for congenital anomalies.

Chest
● To detect pulmonary disorders, including pneumonia, atelectasis, pneumothorax, pulmonary bullae, and tumors
● To look for mediastinal abnormalities, such as tumors, and cardiac disease
● To determine the location and size of a lesion within the chest
● To identify abnormal structures and obstructions, including phleboliths, abnormal gas or fecal collection, and soft-tissue masses, before performing tests that call for instillation of radiopaque dye.

Kidneys, ureters, and bladder
● To evaluate the size, structure, and position of the kidneys
● To screen for abnormalities, such as calcifications, in this region.

Assisting with a portable chest X-ray

When you need to assist with a portable chest X-ray, follow these steps.

Before the procedure
Explain to the patient that a chest X-ray will be performed at the bedside. Tell him that it will be similar to a chest X-ray performed in the radiology department except that he'll have a film plate behind his back. Advise him that the technician will tell him to hold his breath while the X-ray is being taken.

During the procedure
When the technician arrives with the portable X-ray equipment, make sure that nothing is lying on the patient's chest. Move I.V. and arterial lines to the side. Remove any chest electrodes, safety pins, or other metal objects so they won't interfere with the X-ray.

Place the patient in high Fowler's position, and help the technician put the X-ray film plate behind the patient's back. You may have to help the patient lean forward while the film plate is being positioned.

Then help the patient sit so his back makes even contact with the film plate. You may have to stay with him during the procedure to help him maintain his position. If you must stay with him, wear a lead apron. (Lead gloves are also used in some institutions for further protection.) If you're pregnant, don't stay with the patient.

After the procedure
As soon as the technician takes the X-ray, help him remove the film plate from behind the patient's back.

If necessary, reapply chest electrodes. Also, help the patient assume a more comfortable position and make sure any I.V. or arterial lines are intact and working properly.

Abdomen
● To detect gas patterns and loops of dilated bowel to aid in diagnosing GI obstructions and perforations.

Skeleton
● To detect fractures
● To help detect bone tumors
● To assess degenerative conditions
● To detect osteomyelitis.

Procedure-related nursing care
Besides performing the nursing care discussed in the chapter introduction, take the following specific measures. Tell the patient receiving head and neck X-rays that some of the positions he'll have to assume may be uncomfortable. If you're present for the procedure, help him into the various positions for the X-rays as necessary (see *Positioning for a routine skull series*). Leave the room or immediate area when the X-ray is taken to avoid radiation exposure. If you must stay in the area, wear a lead apron or protective clothing.

Normal results
The X-ray should show normal structures for the patient's age.

Abnormal results
Findings vary with the area examined.

Head and neck. The films may reveal fractures of the vault or base of the skull, although basilar fractures may not show up on the film. X-rays may also show congenital anomalies; increased ICP; calcification from osteomyelitis; chronic subdural hematomas; bone changes from metabolic disorders, such as acromegaly or Paget's disease; skull tumors; brain tumors containing calcium; or midline shifting of the calcified pineal gland caused by a space-occupying lesion.

Positioning for a routine skull series

Right and left lateral views
The patient lies with his cheek on the tabletop and the sagittal plane parallel to the tabletop and the film. He rests his chin and neck on his clenched fist or a folded towel. (Each view should show both halves of the mandible directly superimposed.)

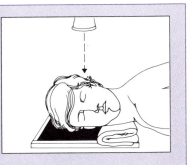

Anteroposterior (Towne's) view
The patient lies supine, with his chin flexed toward the neck. This brings the canthomeatal line perpendicular to the tabletop and the film. The X-ray beam is angled 30 degrees toward the feet.

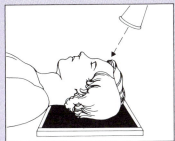

Posteroanterior (Caldwell) view
The patient lies prone (he may support his chin with his fist or a folded towel). The sagittal plane and the canthomeatal line are perpendicular to the tabletop and the film. The X-ray beam is angled 15 degrees toward the feet.

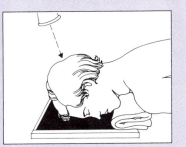

Axial (base) view
The patient lies prone, with his chin fully extended and his face perpendicular to his body. This causes the canthomeatal line to lie parallel to the tabletop and the film.

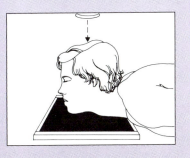

Implications of chest X-rays

STRUCTURE AND NORMAL FINDINGS	ABNORMAL FINDINGS	POSSIBLE CAUSES
Trachea Visible midline in anterior mediastinal cavity; translucent tubelike appearance	• Deviation from midline • Narrowing, with hourglass appearance and deviation to one side	• Tension pneumothorax, atelectasis, pleural effusion, consolidation, mediastinal nodes, or, in children, enlarged thymus • Substernal thyroid
Heart Visible in anterior left mediastinal cavity; solid appearance because of blood contents; edges that may appear clear against surrounding air density of lung	• Position shift • Hypertrophy of the heart's right side • Cardiac borders obscured by varying densities ("shaggy heart")	• Atelectasis • Cor pulmonale or congestive heart failure • Cystic fibrosis
Aortic knob Formed by arch of aorta	• Solid densities (a sign of calcifications) or tortuous shape	• Atherosclerosis
Mediastinum Visible as space between lungs; has shadowy appearance that widens at hilum of lungs	• Deviation from normal position • Gross widening	• Pleural effusion or tumor, fibrosis, or collapsed lung • Neoplasms of esophagus, bronchi, lungs, thyroid, thymus, peripheral nerves, or lymphoid tissue; aortic aneurysm; mediastinitis; or cor pulmonale
Ribs Visible as thoracic cavity encasement	• Break or misalignment • Widening of intercostal spaces	• Fractured sternum or ribs • Emphysema
Spine Visible midline in posterior chest; straight, bony structure	• Spinal curvature • Break or misalignment	• Scoliosis or kyphosis • Fractures
Clavicles Visible in upper thorax; appear intact and equidistant in properly centered X-ray films	• Break or misalignment	• Fractures

Implications of chest X-rays *(continued)*

STRUCTURE AND NORMAL FINDINGS	ABNORMAL FINDINGS	POSSIBLE CAUSES
Hila Visible above heart, where pulmonary vessels and bronchi join lungs; appear small, white, and equally dense	• Shift to one side • Accentuated shadows	• Atelectasis • Emphysema, pulmonary abscess, tumor, or enlarged lymph nodes
Mainstem bronchus Visible as part of hila; trans-lucent tubelike appearance	• Spherical or oval density within bronchus	• Bronchogenic cyst
Bronchi Usually not visible	• Visible	• Bronchial pneumonia
Lung fields Usually not visible through-out, except for blood vessels	• Visible • Irregular, patchy densities	• Atelectasis • Resolving pneumonia, silicosis, fibrosis, or metastatic neoplasm
Hemidiaphragm Visible as rounded structure, with right side ⅜" to ¾" (1 to 2 cm) higher than left	• Elevation of diaphragm • Flattening of diaphragm • Unilateral elevation of either side • Unilateral elevation of left side	• Active tuberculosis, pneumonia, pleurisy, acute bronchitis, active disease of the abdominal viscera, bilateral phrenic nerve involvement, or atelectasis • Asthma or emphysema • Possible unilateral phrenic nerve paresis • Gas distention of stomach, splenic flexure of colon, free air in abdomen, or perforated ulcer (rare)

Chest. Chest X-rays can reveal various disorders. (See *Implications of chest X-rays.*)

Kidneys, ureters, and bladder.
X-rays may disclose kidney enlargement or atrophy, kidney displacement (from a retroperitoneal tumor, for example), absence of a kidney, abnormal kidney location or shape (from congenital anomalies), urinary calculi, vascular calcification, cystic tumors, fecaliths, phleboliths, or foreign bodies.

Abdomen. A flat plate of the abdomen may show abdominal masses, ascites, small-bowel obstruction, abdominal tissue trauma, or calcification of the large blood vessels.

Skeleton. X-ray films may show fractures, osteomyelitis, or degenerative conditions.

Nursing implications of abnormal results
If plain X-ray films suggest a structural abnormality, anticipate further

tests, such as a CT scan, nuclear scan, or biopsy, and prepare the patient as ordered.

If skeletal X-rays confirm a fracture or bone degeneration, prepare the patient as ordered for surgery or application of a cast, a brace, or traction.

Upper GI and small-bowel series

The upper GI and small-bowel series allows fluoroscopic examination of the esophagus, stomach, and small intestine after the patient ingests a contrast agent, usually barium sulfate. (See *Types of contrast media*.) As the barium sulfate passes through the digestive tract, fluoroscopy shows peristalsis and the mucosal contours of the respective organs, and spot films record significant findings.

This test is called for in patients with upper GI signs and symptoms (difficulty swallowing, regurgitation, burning or gnawing epigastric pain), indications of small-bowel disease (diarrhea, weight loss), and signs of GI bleeding (hematemesis, melena). Although this test can detect various mucosal abnormalities, it's commonly followed by a biopsy to rule out cancer or distinguish specific inflammatory diseases.

Because retained barium clouds anatomic detail on X-ray films, this test should be done after a barium enema or routine radiography.

Purpose
• To detect lesions, obstructions, hiatal hernia, diverticula, and varices
• To help diagnose strictures, ulcers, tumors, regional enteritis, and malabsorption syndrome
• To help detect motility disorders.

Procedure-related nursing care
Besides performing the nursing care discussed in the chapter introduction, take the following specific measures.

Before the procedure. Tell the patient he'll lie on an X-ray table that rotates into vertical, semivertical, and horizontal positions. Explain

Types of contrast media

For most GI radiographic tests, the radiologist will choose either barium sulfate or diatrizoate meglumine (Gastrografin) as the contrast medium.

Barium sulfate
Barium sulfate is usually preferred because it shows mucosal detail more clearly and poses a smaller risk of pulmonary edema if accidentally aspirated. The specific barium sulfate preparation depends on the area to be examined and whether the doctor orders a single- or double-contrast test.

Gastrografin
In cases of suspected perforation—especially peritoneal perforation—Gastrografin is preferred. Water-soluble and rapidly reabsorbed, it can leak into the peritoneal cavity without causing problems. Because of this, a doctor will use it first to check for perforation. If none exists, he'll use barium sulfate.

that he'll be secured to the table and that he'll be helped to lie on his back, on his side, and face down, as necessary. Advise him that he may have his abdomen compressed to separate overlapping bowel loops.

Tell him not to eat, drink, or smoke after midnight the night before the test (or for 8 hours before the test). As ordered, withhold most oral medications after midnight. You'll need to withhold anticholinergics and narcotics for 24 hours before the procedure because they affect small-intestinal motility.

Describe the milk-shake consistency and chalky taste of the barium mixture. Warn the patient that although the mixture is flavored, he may not like the taste. Just before the procedure, have him put on a hospital gown without snap closures.

During the procedure. If you're present during the procedure, help the patient assume the various positions for the X-ray as necessary, and provide emotional support.

After the procedure. Make sure the doctor hasn't ordered more X-rays before you allow the patient to have food, fluids, or oral medications.

Tell the patient his stool will look light-colored for 24 to 72 hours after the procedure. Record a description of any stool passed by the patient in the hospital. Since barium retention can cause intestinal obstruction or fecal impaction, encourage the patient to drink extra water — six to eight glasses a day — if he can tolerate the increased fluid intake. Let the doctor know if the patient doesn't pass the barium within 2 or 3 days.

Have the patient rest in bed because this procedure exhausts most patients.

Normal results
The esophagus, stomach, and small intestine should be normal in size and shape. Peristalsis should be normal.

Abnormal results
X-ray studies of the esophagus may reveal strictures, tumors, hiatal hernia, diverticula, varices, ulcers, or achalasia. X-rays of the stomach may show tumors, polyps, ulcers, gastritis, pyloric stenosis, or perforation. Films of the small intestine may disclose regional enteritis, malabsorption syndrome, or tumors.

Nursing implications of abnormal results
If the test results indicate an upper GI disorder, prepare the patient for further testing, as ordered — for instance, the patient will need a biopsy if the test results suggest a tumor. Teach the patient about the recommended treatment plan.

Suggested readings

April, E.W. *Anatomy,* 2nd ed. New York: John Wiley & Sons, 1990.
Corbett, J.V. *Laboratory Tests and Diagnostic Procedures with Nursing Diagnoses,* 2nd ed. Norwalk, Conn.: Appleton & Lange, 1987.
Diagnostics, 2nd ed. Nurse's Reference Library. Springhouse, Pa.: Springhouse Corp., 1987.
Kee, J.L. *Laboratory and Diagnostic Tests with Nursing Implications,* 3rd ed. Norwalk, Conn.: Appleton & Lange, 1990.
Speicher, C.E. *The Right Test: A Physician's Guide to Laboratory Medicine.* Philadelphia: W.B. Saunders Co., 1989.

5

NUCLEAR SCANS

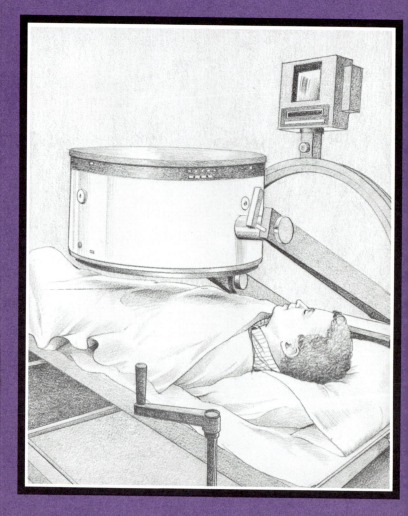

Commonly referred to as scintiscans, scintigraphy, or radionuclide imaging, nuclear scans are based on the principle that specific pathologic conditions will alter the normal distribution of a radioactive tracer. Though each scan uses a particular type of tracer, all nuclear scans work much the same way. The patient is given a tracer, and an imaging device such as a gamma scintillation camera or rectilinear scanner records its distribution.

How nuclear scanning works

Before any scan, the patient receives the tracer—usually intravenously or through a lumbar puncture, although some tracers can be inhaled or taken orally. Once the tracer reaches and concentrates in the appropriate tissue, scanning can begin.

The imaging device maps the distribution of emitted radioactivity and produces an image of the organ on a screen. Areas where the radioactive tracer is distributed equally appear gray. Darker areas, called hot spots, reflect increased uptake of the tracer, and lighter areas, or cold spots, reflect decreased uptake.

These images allow a detailed study of physiologic processes, such as blood flow and excretion. They also provide anatomic information, although other tests, such as computed tomography and ultrasonography, can produce higher-resolution images. Positron emission tomography, a variation of nuclear imaging, provides functional images of biochemical changes. (For more information, see *Positron emission tomography*.)

Risks of nuclear scanning

Like radiographic studies, nuclear scans pose a radiation risk. But because the radioactive tracers have

Positron emission tomography

A form of nuclear computed tomography, positron emission tomography (PET) creates cross-sectional images based on the biochemical and physiologic characteristics of the tissue being scanned. Unlike ultrasonography, computed tomography, and magnetic resonance imaging, which produce only structural images, PET also provides functional images of the biochemical changes that occur in the tissue.

PET scanning requires positron-emitting isotopes, a positron scanner, and a computer to reconstruct the cross-sectional images. The isotopes emit pairs of gamma rays, which the scanner detects. The scanner then relays the information to the computer, which in turn converts this information into an image.

PET helps detect neuropsychiatric problems (Alzheimer's and Parkinson's disease, multiple sclerosis, amyotrophic lateral sclerosis, Huntington's chorea, complex partial seizures, schizophrenia, bipolar affective disorder, and stroke) and cardiac problems (ischemic heart disease). It also allows a doctor to detect and grade malignant tumors.

short half-lives, nuclear scanning usually poses less risk than an X-ray. Still, a pregnant or breast-feeding woman should usually wait to have a nuclear scan.

The radionuclides used also pose the risk of a hypersensitivity reaction, although such reactions rarely occur. But as a precaution, you should check for a history of allergic reactions.

Procedure-related nursing care

The following nursing care measures apply to all nuclear scans covered in this chapter. As part of the discussion of each nuclear scan, you'll also find specific nursing care considerations.

Always explain the purpose of the test to the patient and describe the procedure. Tell him when and how he'll receive the radioactive tracer and where he'll go to receive the scan — usually the nuclear medicine department. Reassure him that the tracer poses little radioactive risk and that the scanning procedure won't cause any pain.

Tell the patient he'll need to follow directions carefully. He'll be told, for instance, to keep still during the scanning procedure to prevent the image from blurring. If the patient doesn't follow such directions, he may have to undergo the test again.

Tell a pregnant woman or a woman who's breast-feeding that the doctor may postpone the scan to protect the fetus or child from radiation exposure. A woman may instead stop breast-feeding for a specific time period before and after the scan, so the radionuclide doesn't collect in her breast milk.

Make sure the patient or a responsible family member signs an informed consent form before a procedure that calls for an injection or any other invasive procedure.

Just before the scan, tell the patient to remove jewelry, dentures, and other metal objects that might interfere with the scan.

After the procedure, encourage the patient to drink extra fluids, unless contraindicated. This helps eliminate the radioactive tracer. Because isotopes pass from the body in urine, tell the patient to flush twice after urinating for the first 24 hours after the scan. Anyone who must handle a urine specimen from the patient should follow universal precautions during this period.

Bone scan

Used mainly to detect lesions, a bone scan (radionuclide bone imaging) provides images of the skeleton after I.V. injection of a radioactive tracer compound. This tracer collects in bone tissue, concentrating at sites of abnormal metabolism. Bone scanning allows a doctor to detect a lesion months before an X-ray would reveal it.

Purpose
• To detect and locate malignant bone lesions or metastases when radiographic findings appear normal but cancer is confirmed or suspected
• To detect occult bone trauma from pathologic fractures
• To monitor degenerative bone disorders
• To detect infection.

Procedure-related nursing care
Besides performing the nursing care discussed in the chapter introduction, take the following specific measures. Before the scan, tell the patient he'll receive an I.V. injection of a radioactive agent. Explain that he'll assume various positions on a scanner table and that the test usually takes about an hour, although it may take longer if the doctor needs extra pictures.

If the doctor ordered the bone scan to diagnose cancer, provide emotional support as needed. If he ordered it to monitor the spread of a cancer or degenerative bone disease, administer an analgesic, as ordered, to help keep the patient as comfortable as possible when changing positions or holding the same position for an extended period during the test.

Because the patient must drink several glasses of water or tea immediately before scanning begins (about 1 to 3 hours after injection of the tracer), advise him to drink as little as possible for several hours before the injection. Tell him to void before he's positioned on the scanner table.

Normal results

Normally, the tracer concentrates in bone tissue at sites of new bone formation or increased metabolism — for instance, in the epiphyses of growing bone.

Abnormal results

Hot spots revealed by a scan can help identify various types of bone cancer, infection, fractures, and other disorders when interpreted in light of the patient's medical and surgical history, X-rays, and other laboratory tests.

Nursing implications of abnormal results

When the results indicate malignant bone metastases or a degenerative disease, provide emotional support for the patient and his family. Make sure you understand the therapeutic plan so you can explain it to them.

Also, try to make the patient as comfortable as possible. Refer him to support groups that might help him cope with his diagnosis.

Cardiac blood pool imaging

Cardiac blood pool imaging primarily evaluates regional and global ventricular performance after I.V. injection of human serum albumin or red blood cells (RBCs) tagged with a radioisotope or a radiopaque dye that attaches to the RBCs.

This test — also called cardiac blood pool scanning, nuclear ventriculography, and multigated nuclear ventriculography — can take several forms. In first-pass imaging, a scintillation camera records the radioactivity emitted by the tracer as it passes through the right atrium and ventricle to the pulmonary artery and veins and then through the left atrium and ventricle. The portion of tracer ejected by the left ventricle during each heartbeat can be calculated to determine the ejection fraction. The test also helps determine the presence and size of intracardiac shunts.

Gated cardiac blood pool imaging, performed after first-pass imaging or as a separate test, usually uses signals from an electrocardiogram (ECG) to trigger the scintillation camera. In two-frame gated imaging, the camera records left ventricular end-systole and end-diastole for 500 to 1,000 cardiac cycles. When superimposed, these gated images allow a clinician to assess left ventricular contractions and find areas of dyskinesia or akinesia. In multiple-gated acquisition (MUGA) scanning, the camera records 14 to 64 points of a single cardiac cycle. The resulting sequential images can then be studied like a motion picture to evaluate regional wall motion and determine the ejection fraction and other indices of cardiac function.

Two variations of the MUGA test assess the heart's function in response to stimulation. The stress MUGA test is performed at rest and after exercise to detect changes in the ejection fraction and cardiac output. In the nitro MUGA test, the scintillation camera records points in the cardiac cycle after the patient receives sublingual nitroglycerin. This test assesses the nitroglycerin's effect on ventricular function.

Purpose
• To evaluate ventricular function
• To detect aneurysms of the left ventricle and other myocardial wall-motion abnormalities (areas of akinesia or dyskinesia)
• To detect intracardiac shunting
• To determine the extent of muscle impairment after a myocardial infarction.

Procedure-related nursing care
Besides performing the nursing care discussed in the chapter introduction, take the following specific measures. Tell the patient that ECG electrodes will be placed on his chest and that he'll receive an I.V. injection of a radioactive agent. Warn him that he may find the needle puncture uncomfortable. Explain, too, that he'll need to remain silent and motionless during imaging, unless otherwise instructed.

Encourage him to rest and avoid heavy meals for about a day before the test. If he's having the stress MUGA test, make sure he has socks and snug-fitting shoes for the test. Tell an outpatient to put on comfortable clothing and snug-fitting shoes, such as sneakers or running shoes.

Normal results
Normally, the left ventricle contracts symmetrically, and the isotope appears evenly distributed in the scans. The normal ejection fraction ranges from 55% to 65%.

Abnormal results
The test may reveal left ventricular abnormalities resulting from coronary artery disease as well as aneurysms of the left ventricle, cardiomyopathy, congestive heart failure, or intracardiac shunting.

Nursing implications of abnormal results
If the test results indicate impaired ventricular function, explain the prescribed medical or surgical treatment to the patient. If his ventricular function is seriously impaired, explain the importance of decreasing his heart's work load by avoiding stressful situations and decreasing his physical activity.

Cisternography

For this test, a radioactive tracer is injected into the patient's lumbar subarachnoid space. The tracer then travels with the cerebrospinal fluid (CSF), so a scanner can produce an image of CSF flow through the brain's cistern and ventricles.

The tracer should outline the complete path of the CSF within 24 hours. (See *Tracing normal CSF circulation.*) If it doesn't, the cisternogram confirms an abnormality, such as ventricular entry from hydrocephalus.

You may also hear the cisternogram called a RISA scan, a radionuclide scan of the cisterns and ventricles of the brain, or a CSF flow scan.

Purpose
• To diagnose hydrocephalus
• To detect a CSF leak.

Procedure-related nursing care
Besides performing the nursing care discussed in the chapter introduction, take the following specific measures.

Tell the patient (or his parents if

Tracing normal CSF circulation

Cerebrospinal fluid (CSF) is produced in the choroid plexus, capillary networks in the brain's lateral, third, and fourth ventricles. The CSF that filters into the lateral ventricles flows through the foramen of Monro into the third ventricle. CSF from the lateral and the third ventricles then flows through the aqueduct of Sylvius into the fourth ventricle. And CSF from the lateral, third, and fourth ventricles flows through the foramina of Luschka and Magendie to the subarachnoid space.

In the subarachnoid space, which surrounds the entire brain and spinal cord, the fluid passes under the base of the brain, upward over the brain's upper surface, and down around the spinal cord. When CSF reaches the arachnoid villi, the venous sinuses absorb the CSF into the venous blood.

Normally, the amount of CSF produced (500 to 800 ml/day) equals the amount absorbed. The average amount circulating at one time is 125 to 175 ml.

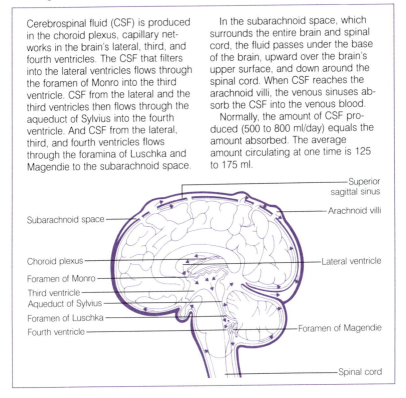

the patient is an infant) that the doctor will perform a lumbar puncture and inject a radioactive tracer. Then the patient will return to his room and lie flat for 4 to 6 hours to help prevent a headache from the puncture and to allow the tracer to circulate. After that, a scan will be taken. He'll have another scan 24 hours after the injection, and possibly a third and fourth scan 48 and 72 hours after the injection. Explain that he'll need to lie flat during the scanning.

After the procedure, make sure the patient receives extra fluids and lies flat, as ordered, to help prevent

a headache from the lumbar puncture.

Normal results
The scan should show a normal CSF flow into the cisterns and the ventricles.

Abnormal results
The scan may detect normal-pressure, communicating, or external obstructive hydrocephalus, or a CSF leak.

Nursing implications of abnormal results
If the test results indicate hydro-

cephalus, make sure you understand the treatment plan so you can explain it to the patient or his parents and answer any questions. If necessary, prepare the patient for surgery.

Gallbladder scan

Also called cholescintigraphy or radionuclide imaging of hepatobiliary excretion, the gallbladder scan uses a gamma scintillation camera to take a series of images after I.V. injection of a radioactive tracer. The hepatobiliary system rapidly excretes the tracer, so the serial images show radioactivity not only in the gallbladder, but also in the liver, bile ducts, and duodenum. In a patient with severe hepatocellular disease, images of the gallbladder may be taken 6 to 48 hours after injection to give the diseased gallbladder a longer opportunity to take up the tracer.

Quicker and more accurate than oral cholecystography, the gallbladder scan is rapidly becoming the test of choice for detecting gallbladder disease.

Purpose
• To help diagnose cholecystitis, cholelithiasis, biliary obstruction, biliary tract leaks, biliary anomalies, liver disease, and cancer of the hepatobiliary system
• To determine bile-enteric patency after diversionary procedures
• To identify cystic duct remnants after cholecystectomy
• To determine liver rejection after transplantation.

Procedure-related nursing care
Besides performing the nursing care

discussed in the chapter introduction, take the following specific measures. Tell the patient he'll receive an I.V. dose of a radioactive agent right before the procedure. Ask him if he's ever had gallbladder or liver disease, or gallbladder surgery. If so, tell the doctor and radiologist.

Restrict food and fluid intake for at least 2 — preferably 4 — hours before the test.

Normal results
The liver, gallbladder, and biliary tract should have normal size, shape, and function.

Abnormal results
The scan may identify acute, chronic, or acalculous cholecystitis; cholelithiasis; cholestasis resulting from hepatocellular disease or bile duct obstruction; bile leaks or fistulas; biliary atresia; liver metastases; or liver rejection after transplantation.

Nursing implications of abnormal results
If the test results indicate acute gallbladder disease, make sure the patient rests and try to make him as comfortable as possible. If necessary, prepare him for surgery.

Gallium scanning

In this test, a gamma scintillation camera or rectilinear scanner scans the entire body, usually 24 to 48 hours after I.V. injection of radioactive gallium citrate. Occasionally, the scan takes place 72 hours after the injection. For a patient with acute inflammatory disease, the doctor may order the scan 4 to 6 hours after the injection.

Besides the liver, spleen, bones, and large bowel, certain neoplasms and inflammatory lesions also take up the gallium. However, several neoplasms and a few inflammatory lesions don't take it up, and gallium has an affinity for both benign and malignant neoplasms. Because of this drawback, an exact diagnosis requires further tests, such as computed tomography.

Still, gallium scanning can help pinpoint the site of a disease (usually a cancer) that other tests haven't clearly defined. It also can clarify focal hepatic defects when liver-spleen scanning and ultrasonography prove inconclusive. Plus, the test can be used to evaluate suspected bronchogenic carcinoma when a sputum culture proves positive for cancer but other tests are normal, or when the patient has hydrothorax, preventing the use of bronchoscopy.

Purpose
• To detect primary or metastatic neoplasms and inflammatory lesions
• To evaluate malignant lymphoma and identify recurrent tumors after chemotherapy or radiation therapy
• To clarify focal defects in the liver
• To evaluate bronchogenic carcinoma.

Procedure-related nursing care
Besides performing the nursing care discussed in the chapter introduction, take the following specific measures. Tell the patient that he'll receive an I.V. injection of radioactive gallium 24 to 48 hours before the scan. If a gamma scintillation camera is used, explain that, although the uptake probe and detector head may touch his skin, he won't feel any discomfort. If a rectilinear scanner is used, tell the patient that it makes a soft, irregular clicking noise as it registers the radiation emissions. Administer a laxative or cleansing enema or both, as ordered, just before the scan.

If the test suggests bowel disease and the patient needs further scans, give a cleansing enema, as ordered, before the next series of scans.

Normal results
Gallium activity is normally demonstrated in the liver, spleen, bones, and large bowel.

Abnormal results
Gallium scanning may reveal inflammatory lesions — either discrete abscesses or diffuse infiltration, such as bacterial peritonitis. It can also reveal inflammatory diseases (such as sarcoidosis) and cancers, including various sarcomas, Wilms' tumor, neuroblastomas, and carcinomas of the kidney, uterus, vagina, stomach, and testes. Scanning can indicate the extent of Hodgkin's disease and non-Hodgkin's lymphoma.

Nursing implications of abnormal results
If the test results indicate cancer, provide emotional support for the patient and his family. Describe the treatment and answer any questions they have.

If the test results indicate an inflammation, help the patient rest and explain the treatment regimen to him. Make sure he and his family understand the difference between inflammation and cancer.

Liver-spleen scan

This nuclear scan of the liver and spleen serves as one of the most reliable screening tests for hepatocel-

Understanding liver flow studies

Unlike a liver-spleen scan, which produces static images, liver flow studies (dynamic scintigraphy) record the stages of perfusion in rapid sequence. Because these studies demonstrate the vascularity of focal defects, they can help differentiate cysts, abscesses, tumors, and metastases.

Cysts and abscesses, which don't have blood vessels, can't take up the radionuclide at all and appear as cold spots. Hemangiomas, which have enlarged vessels, take up the radionuclide easily and show up as hot spots. Tumors and metastases have variable vascularity, making them difficult to evaluate. Vascular metastases, for instance, may appear hot, but most metastases don't take up much radionuclide. And hepatomas may show up as hot spots, or they may be hard to distinguish from the surrounding parenchyma.

lular disease, hepatic metastases, and focal defects, such as tumors, cysts, and abscesses. But the test does have some drawbacks. It shows focal defects nonspecifically as cold spots, and it may not detect lesions smaller than ¾″ (2 cm) in diameter. It may also miss early hepatocellular disease.

Liver-spleen scanning commonly requires confirmation by ultrasonography, computed tomography, gallium scanning, biopsy, or liver flow studies (see *Understanding liver flow studies*). After metastasis has been confirmed, serial liver-spleen studies can help evaluate the effectiveness of therapy.

Purpose
• To screen for hepatic metastases and hepatocellular diseases, such as cirrhosis and hepatitis

• To detect focal disease in the liver and spleen
• To demonstrate hepatomegaly, splenomegaly, and splenic infarctions
• To assess the condition of the liver and spleen after abdominal trauma
• To evaluate the effectiveness of therapy.

Procedure-related nursing care
Besides performing the nursing care discussed in the chapter introduction, tell the patient he'll receive a small I.V. injection of a radioactive agent 10 to 15 minutes before the scan. Also, explain that he'll have to assume various positions as the camera scans his abdomen.

Normal results
The liver and spleen should appear normal in size, shape, and position. But the liver, which has various normal indentations and impressions, such as the gallbladder fossa and falciform ligament, won't distribute the radioactive agent as uniformly as the spleen, and its indentations may mimic focal disease.

Abnormal results
This scan may show hepatocellular disease (hepatitis or cirrhosis), portal hypertension, obstruction of the superior vena cava, Budd-Chiari syndrome, splenic infarction, and focal defects (cysts, abscesses, primary tumors, metastases, and hematoma) caused by hepatic or splenic disorders.

Nursing implications of abnormal results
If the test results indicate cirrhosis, prepare the patient for further tests, including liver enzyme, serum electrolyte, and plasma ammonia tests. He'll also need a liver biopsy to confirm the diagnosis.

If the test results point to cancer or another serious disorder, provide emotional support. Explain the treatment plan to the patient and answer any questions he may have.

Lung perfusion scan

The lung perfusion scan (lung scintiscan) produces an image of pulmonary blood flow after I.V. injection of a radionuclide. When performed with a ventilation scan, this test allows a doctor to assess a patient's ventilation-perfusion patterns. (See *Ventilation scan.*) The lung perfusion scan can also detect pulmonary vascular obstructions, such as pulmonary emboli, although a ventilation scan confirms the diagnosis.

Purpose
• To assess lung perfusion
• To detect pulmonary emboli
• To evaluate the pulmonary function of a preoperative patient with marginal lung reserves.

Procedure-related nursing care
Besides performing the nursing care discussed in the chapter introduction, inform the patient that he'll have the scan right after receiving an I.V. injection of a radioactive tracer.

Normal results
A normal scan shows a uniform uptake pattern of the radionuclide, a sign of normal pulmonary blood flow.

Abnormal results
Cold spots — areas of low uptake — indicate poor perfusion, suggesting a problem such as an embolus. Decreased regional blood flow that occurs without vessel obstruction may signal pneumonitis.

Ventilation scan

Performed with a lung perfusion scan, a ventilation scan helps distinguish between parenchymal disease, such as bronchogenic carcinoma, and conditions caused by vascular abnormalities, such as pulmonary emboli. Whereas parenchymal disease causes an abnormal ventilation scan, a pulmonary embolus affects only perfusion, not ventilation.

How the test works
After the patient inhales air mixed with radioactive gas, the scan outlines areas of the lung that are ventilated. It records gas distribution over three phases: during the buildup of radioactive gas (wash-in phase), after the patient rebreathes from a bag and the radioactivity reaches a steady level (equilibrium phase), and after he exhales the radioactive gas from his lungs (wash-out phase).

What the results mean
Normally, the radioactive gas will be distributed equally in both lungs. Areas of low radioactivity indicate decreased ventilation. Unequal gas distribution in both lungs stems from poor ventilation or an airway obstruction. Abnormal ventilation within areas of consolidation signals parenchymal disease, such as pneumonia. Regional hypoventilation usually results from excessive smoking or chronic obstructive pulmonary disease.

Nursing implications of abnormal results
If the test results suggest a pulmonary embolus, anticipate a ventilation scan to confirm the diagnosis. Administer oxygen, anticoagulant therapy, and analgesics, as ordered.

Renal scan

This scan can be used to evaluate the function of one or both kidneys. When performed in conjunction with radionuclide renography — a test that provides a curve illustrating the uptake, transit, and excretion time of a radioactive tracer — a renal scan can give further information about renal perfusion. A renal scan can also take the place of I.V. pyelography when a patient has a hypersensitivity to contrast agents.

Purpose
• To detect or rule out masses, trauma, inflammation, and infection
• To check the patency of the urinary system
• To assess kidney function
• To help rule out a renovascular cause for hypertension
• To evaluate a renal transplant.

Procedure-related nursing care
Besides performing the nursing care discussed in the chapter introduction, tell the patient he'll receive the scan right after I.V. injection of a radioactive agent.

Normal results
The tracer should disperse uniformly throughout both kidneys, revealing normal size, shape, position, and function.

Abnormal results
The scan may reveal space-occupying lesions, such as masses within the kidney; decreased uptake in one or both kidneys; dilation of the collecting system of one of the kidneys, indicating an obstruction; decreased kidney function; or organ rejection after a transplant.

Nursing implications of abnormal results
If the test results reveal abnormal kidney function, prepare the patient for further studies as necessary. Make sure you understand the treatment plan so you can explain it to the patient.

Scrotal scan

Helpful in detecting — although not in diagnosing — testicular abnormalities, this test uses a scanning camera to take images of the testes and scrotum after I.V. injection of a radioactive tracer. The scrotal scan (also called a testicular scan or radionuclide scan of the scrotum or testes) shows abnormalities as either cold or hot spots. Cold spots may signal a hydrocele; hot spots may signal a malignant tumor, an abscess, or epididymitis. Testicular torsion results in an uneven flow and distribution of the radionuclide.

Purpose
• To detect or rule out testicular torsion
• To detect an abnormality of the testes
• To detect or rule out epididymitis.

Procedure-related nursing care
Besides performing the nursing care discussed in the chapter introduction, take the following specific measures. Tell the patient that he'll receive an oral medication — usually potassium perchlorate — before the scan. This will keep the radioactive agent he'll receive from concentrating in his thyroid gland. Also, explain that the agent won't be injected until after he's positioned under the camera.

Normal results
The tracer should flow uniformly throughout the scrotal sac.

Abnormal results
The scan may reveal testicular torsion, hydrocele, a malignant tumor, an abscess, or epididymitis.

Nursing implications of abnormal results
If the test results suggest testicular cancer, provide the patient with emotional support and prepare him for further testing, such as a biopsy, to confirm the diagnosis. If results indicate testicular torsion, prepare him for surgery. For epididymitis, follow the prescribed medical treatment.

Thyroid scan

Usually recommended after the discovery of a palpable mass, an enlarged gland, or an asymmetrical goiter, this test consists of administering a radioisotope — typically an iodine isotope — then scanning the thyroid gland. Also called radionuclide thyroid imaging, the thyroid scan is usually performed along with measurements of serum triiodothyronine (T_3) and serum thyroxine (T_4) levels, and the thyroid uptake test.

If the scan shows areas of increased uptake, or hot spots, a T_3 thyroid suppression test usually follows to determine whether these areas are autonomous or a sign of pituitary overcompensation. (See *T_3 thyroid suppression test.*)

If cold spots appear, thyroid ultrasonography can rule out cysts, and fine-needle aspiration and biopsy can rule out cancer.

T_3 thyroid suppression test

The T_3 thyroid suppression test helps determine whether areas of excessive iodine uptake in the thyroid (hot spots) are autonomous, as in some cases of Graves' disease, or reflect pituitary overcompensation, as in iodine-deficient goiter.

Autonomous hot spots function independently of pituitary control. But hot spots caused by iodine deficiency stem from reduced T_4 production, which decreases T_3 production and increases thyroid-stimulating hormone (TSH) production. Increased TSH production, in turn, overstimulates the thyroid and causes excessive iodine uptake.

How the test works
After a baseline reading of thyroid function is obtained from a radioactive iodine uptake (RAIU) test, the patient receives 100 μg of synthetic T_3 (Cytomel) for 7 days. (Normally, T_3 acts through a negative feedback mechanism to suppress pituitary release of TSH, which in turn decreases thyroid function and iodine uptake.) During the last 2 days of Cytomel administration, RAIU tests are repeated to assess thyroid response.

What the results mean
Suppression of RAIU to at least 50% of baseline indicates that the hot spot is under pituitary control and suggests iodine deficiency as the cause of increased iodine uptake. Failure to suppress RAIU by 50% suggests autonomous thyroid hyperfunction, resulting perhaps from Graves' disease or a toxic thyroid nodule.

Purpose
• To evaluate thyroid function in conjunction with specific thyroid uptake studies
• To assess the size, structure, and position of the thyroid gland.

Interpreting thyroid scan results

CONDITION	FINDINGS	POSSIBLE CAUSES
Hypothyroidism	• Glandular damage or absent gland	Surgical removal of gland, inflammation, radiation, or neoplasm (rare)
Nontoxic goiter	• Enlarged gland • Normal or decreased uptake	Insufficient iodine intake or impaired thyroid hormone synthesis
Myxedema (cretinism in children)	• Normal or slightly reduced gland size • Uniform pattern • Decreased uptake	Defective embryonic development, resulting in congenital absence or underdevelopment of thyroid gland; maternal iodine deficiency
Hyperthyroidism (Graves' disease)	• Enlarged gland • Uniform pattern • Increased uptake	Production of thyroid-stimulating immunoglobulins
Toxic nodular goiter	• Multiple hot spots	Long-standing simple goiter
Hyperfunctioning adenoma	• Solitary hot spot	Adenomatous production of T_3 and T_4, suppressing TSH secretion and producing atrophy of other thyroid tissue
Hypofunctioning adenoma	• Solitary cold spot	Cyst or nonfunctioning nodule
Benign multinodular goiter	• Multiple nodules with variable or no function	Local inflammation or degeneration
Thyroid carcinoma	• Usually a solitary cold spot with occasional or no function	Neoplasm

Procedure-related nursing care

Besides performing the nursing care discussed in the chapter introduction, take the following specific measures. Tell a patient receiving an oral radioactive agent that he'll undergo the scan 24 hours later. Tell a patient receiving an I.V. dose that he'll undergo the scan 20 to 30 minutes later.

Check the patient's history to determine which drugs or foods he may need to discontinue before the test. As ordered, tell the patient to discontinue any thyroid hormone, thyroid hormone antagonist, or iodine preparation (such as Lugol's solution, some types of multivitamins, and cough syrup) 2 to 3 weeks before the test. Tell the patient taking phenothiazine to stop a week before. The patient may also have to avoid iodized salt, salt substitutes, and seafood before the test.

Ask the patient if he has undergone any tests within the past 60 days that used a radiographic contrast agent. Note your findings on the request slip because such agents may interfere with iodine uptake.

Normal results
The thyroid should take up the radioisotope uniformly, demonstrating normal size, shape, position, and function.

Abnormal results
Hot spots indicate hyperfunctioning nodules; cold spots, hypofunctioning nodules. (See *Interpreting thyroid scan results.*)

Nursing implications of abnormal results
If test results indicate a thyroid problem, prepare the patient for further studies, such as thyroid ultrasonography, as ordered. If results suggest a cancer, he'll need a fine-needle thyroid aspiration or a thyroid biopsy.

Suggested readings

Bentley, L.J. "Radionuclide Imaging Techniques in the Diagnosis and Treatment of Coronary Heart Disease," *Focus on Critical Care* 14(6):27-36, December 1987.

Corbett, J.V. *Laboratory Tests and Diagnostic Procedures with Nursing Diagnoses,* 2nd ed. Norwalk, Conn.: Appleton & Lange, 1987.

Diagnostics, 2nd ed. Nurse's Reference Library. Springhouse, Pa.: Springhouse Corp., 1987.

Fischbach, F.T. *A Manual of Laboratory Diagnostic Tests,* 3rd ed. Philadelphia: J.B. Lippincott Co., 1988.

Kee, J.L. *Laboratory and Diagnostic Tests with Nursing Implications,* 3rd ed. Norwalk, Conn.: Appleton & Lange, 1990.

Speicher, C.E. *The Right Test: A Physician's Guide to Laboratory Medicine.* Philadelphia: W.B. Saunders Co., 1989.

6

ULTRASONOGRAPHY

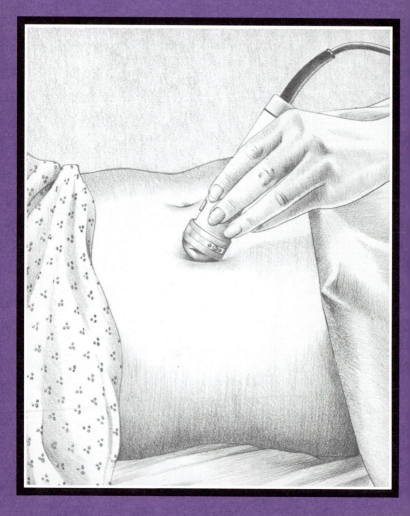

A relatively safe, noninvasive diagnostic procedure, ultrasonography uses high-frequency sound waves to study soft-tissue structures. Ultrasonography can show the size, consistency, and shape of internal structures and can detect such abnormalities as calculi, masses, edema, inflammation, and free fluid. The procedure also can differentiate between cystic and solid masses, outline the boundaries of lesions, show the displacement of adjacent tissues, show motion, and allow continuous viewing of a structure. One type of ultrasonography, Doppler ultrasonography, can detect a fetal heartbeat and evaluate blood flow in the major vessels of the neck, arms, and legs.

How ultrasonography works

During ultrasonography, the examiner presses a transducer against the patient's skin and moves it over the pertinent body area. Applying a coupling agent, such as a conductive gel, eliminates air trapping between the transducer and the skin, promoting good acoustic contact. The transducer converts electrical signals to ultrasonic waves and sends them into the desired area. At the same time, the transducer receives the waves as they bounce back from the structures being examined and converts them into electrical signals again. A computer then transforms these electrical signals into scans, graphs or, in the case of Doppler ultrasonography, audible sounds.

Ultrasound procedures usually are performed in an ultrasound room. However, some procedures may be done at the patient's bedside, if necessary.

Ultrasonography carries only minor disadvantages. For instance, it can't be used to examine bones or air-filled organs, and the study of abdominal and pelvic structures may be obscured by the overlying bowel. The procedure also may be difficult to perform on certain patients. For example, the transducer must be moved carefully over a new surgical incision, and scar tissue can attenuate the ultrasound beam. Ultrasonography also may be difficult in an obese patient because adipose tissue can interfere with sound wave transmission.

Procedure-related nursing care

The following nursing care measures apply to all ultrasound procedures covered in this chapter. As part of the discussion of each procedure, you'll also find specific nursing care considerations.

Explain the procedure and its purpose to the patient. Tell him that the examiner will apply a conductive gel to the appropriate area of his body, then pass a transducer over it. Reassure the patient that the procedure is safe and painless, although he may feel mild pressure as the examiner moves the transducer over the skin. If the patient is pregnant, reassure her that the test won't harm the fetus.

Tell the patient that the procedure usually takes about 30 to 45 minutes. Instruct him to remain still when requested during the procedure; explain that movement can interfere with accurate study results. Also, tell him that he may be asked to change positions so his organs can be seen at different angles. Inform him that dressings at the ultrasound site will be removed, if possible.

Make sure the patient isn't scheduled for a barium enema or an upper GI series before the study. (The high-frequency sound waves can't penetrate barium.)

For routine ultrasound studies,

signed consent isn't necessary. Because the procedure is noninvasive and safe, no special nursing assessment is required afterward. But be sure to remove any remaining conductive gel from the skin and replace any dressings that were removed.

Abdominal aorta ultrasonography

In this procedure, a transducer directs high-frequency sound waves into the abdomen over a wide area from the xiphoid process to the umbilical region. The sound waves, echoing to the transducer from tissues of different densities, are transmitted as electrical impulses and displayed on an oscilloscope or television screen to reveal internal organs, the vertebral column and, most important, the size and course of the abdominal aorta and other major vessels.

This study helps confirm a suspected aortic aneurysm and is the method of choice for determining its diameter. If an aneurysm is detected but surgery won't be performed immediately, ultrasonography will probably be done every 6 months to monitor the size of the aneurysm.

If surgery will be performed, angiography is indicated preoperatively to visualize the extent of atherosclerotic changes and to reveal any anatomic anomalies, such as three renal arteries. It's also indicated when the diagnosis is unclear.

Purpose
• To detect and measure a suspected abdominal aortic aneurysm

• To detect and measure expansion of a known abdominal aortic aneurysm.

Procedure-related nursing care
Besides performing the nursing care discussed in the chapter introduction, take the following specific measures. Instruct the patient to avoid food and fluids for 12 hours before the test to minimize bowel gas and motility. If ordered, administer simethicone to reduce bowel gas.

If the patient has a known aneurysm, reassure him that the sound waves can't cause it to rupture.

After the procedure, instruct the patient to resume his normal diet.

Normal results
In adults, the diameter of a normal abdominal aorta tapers from about 2.5 cm at the diaphragm to about 1.5 cm at the bifurcation. The aorta descends through the retroperitoneal space, anterior to the vertebral column and slightly left of the midline. Its major branches — the celiac trunk, the renal arteries, the superior mesenteric artery, and the common iliac arteries — usually can be well visualized.

Abnormal results
A lumen diameter greater than 4 cm is considered an aneurysm; a diameter greater than 7 cm, an aneurysm with a high risk of rupture.

Nursing implications of abnormal results
If ultrasonography reveals an aneurysm greater than 5 cm in diameter — and if the patient is a good surgical candidate — the doctor typically will recommend surgery. In most cases, surgery also is recommended for a symptomatic patient regardless of the aneurysm's size. If surgery is indicated, prepare the pa-

tient physically and emotionally.

If ultrasonography reveals an aneurysm between 4 and 5 cm in diameter, the doctor may or may not recommend immediate surgery, usually depending on the risk the surgery poses to the patient. If the patient isn't considered a candidate for immediate surgery, stress the importance of careful medical follow-up. Schedule subsequent ultrasound examinations at recommended intervals and teach the patient the signs and symptoms of an impending rupture. Emphasize the need to notify the doctor immediately of any abdominal or back discomfort.

Keep in mind that a patient with a history of symptomatic cardiac or carotid artery disease is at increased risk for myocardial infarction during surgery and the postoperative period.

Doppler ultrasonography

This noninvasive procedure evaluates blood flow in the major veins and arteries of the arms and legs and in the extracranial cerebrovascular system. Developed as an alternative to arteriography and venography, Doppler ultrasonography is quicker, safer, and less costly than invasive tests. Although this procedure has a 95% accuracy rate in detecting arteriovenous disease that significantly impairs blood flow, it may fail to detect mild arteriosclerotic plaques and smaller thrombi and generally fails to detect major calf vein thrombosis.

In Doppler ultrasonography, a hand-held transducer directs high-frequency sound waves to the artery or vein being tested. The sound waves strike moving red blood cells

and are reflected to the transducer at frequencies that correspond to the velocity of blood flow through the vessel. The transducer then amplifies the sound waves to permit direct listening. (See *How the Doppler probe works,* page 144.)

Measuring systolic blood pressure during Doppler ultrasonography helps detect the presence, location, and extent of peripheral arterial occlusive disease. Observing changes in sound wave frequency during respirations helps detect venous occlusive disease because venous blood flow normally fluctuates with respiration. Using compression maneuvers also can help detect venous occlusion as well as occlusion or stenosis of carotid arteries. (For more information, see *Understanding carotid imaging,* page 145.)

Pulse volume recorder testing may be performed in conjunction with Doppler ultrasonography to yield a quantitative recording of changes in blood volume or flow in a limb or an organ.

Purpose
● To aid in diagnosing chronic venous insufficiency and superficial and deep vein thromboses (popliteal, femoral, or iliac)
● To aid in diagnosing peripheral artery disease and arterial occlusion
● To monitor patients who've undergone arterial reconstruction and bypass grafting procedures
● To detect abnormalities of carotid artery blood flow associated with such conditions as aortic stenosis
● To evaluate possible arterial trauma
● To detect a fetal heartbeat.

Procedure-related nursing care
Besides performing the nursing care discussed in the chapter introduction, take the following specific mea-

How the Doppler probe works

The Doppler ultrasonic probe directs high-frequency sound waves through tissue layers. When these waves strike red blood cells (RBCs) moving through the bloodstream, the frequency of the sound waves changes in proportion to the flow velocity of the RBCs. Recording these waves permits the examiner to detect arterial and venous obstruction but not to measure blood flow quantitatively.

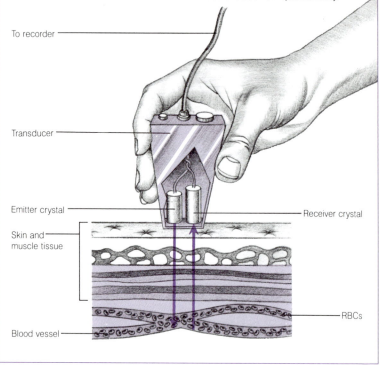

To recorder

Transducer

Emitter crystal

Receiver crystal

Skin and muscle tissue

RBCs

Blood vessel

sures. Explain to the patient that the examiner may ask him to remove all his clothing either above or below the waist, depending on the examination site. If Doppler ultrasonography is being done for peripheral artery evaluation, explain that the procedure also will include blood pressure measurement at several sites along the limb being examined. If the procedure is being done for peripheral vein evaluation, explain that the examiner may perform compression maneuvers to assess vein competence. For evaluation of the leg, inform the patient that he'll be asked to perform Valsalva's maneuver as venous blood flow is recorded.

Normal results

The ratio between ankle systolic pressure and brachial systolic pressure — the ankle-arm pressure index (API), also known as the arterial ischemia index, the ankle-brachial index, or the pedal-brachial index — normally is 1 or greater. Proximal thigh pressure normally is 20 to 30 mm Hg higher than arm pressure, but pressure measurements at sites adjacent to the thigh are similar. In the arms, pressure readings should remain unchanged despite postural changes. Segmental pressures in the limbs should be equal. Audible signals indicate unobstructed venous and arterial blood flow bilaterally.

Abnormal results

An abnormal API is directly proportional to the degree of circulatory impairment. An API of 1 to 0.75 correlates with mild ischemia; 0.75 to 0.5, with claudication; 0.5 to 0.25, with pain at rest; and 0.25 to 0, with pregangrene. Diminished blood flow velocity indicates venous or arterial stenosis or occlusion. An absent venous flow velocity may indicate venous thrombosis.

Nursing implications of abnormal results

Prepare the patient for more definitive diagnostic studies as indicated. If Doppler ultrasonography confirms peripheral vein thrombosis, closely monitor circulation and motor and sensory function in the affected limb. Also, administer anticoagulant and thrombolytic medications, as ordered.

If the results, along with the health history and physical assessment findings, indicate peripheral arterial occlusion, teach the patient the importance of reducing his risk factors, exercising, performing proper foot and leg care, and taking his prescribed medications. When indicated, prepare the patient for percutaneous transluminal angioplasty or for more extensive surgery.

Understanding carotid imaging

This diagnostic test assesses the carotid arteries for occlusive disease. Carotid imaging can detect ulcerating plaques that can't be detected by other methods. Plus, the test can differentiate between total and near-total arterial occlusion.

The procedure does have a disadvantage, though. Intramural calcification prevents sound penetration and may lead to false-positive results.

How carotid imaging works

With the patient supine, the examiner will place the probe on his neck. Then he'll move the probe slowly from the vicinity of the common carotid artery to that of the bifurcation, then to the internal and external carotids. The examiner may use either a real-time imager or a pulsed Doppler ultrasonic flow transducer.

Real-time imaging uses the echo technique, which permits visualization of the carotid artery. Thus, a Doppler signal can be directed to specific points along the vessel. The audio signal is then evaluated.

The pulsed Doppler technique uses a transducer with a range-gating system that allows alternate transmission and reception of ultrasonic signals. The sound reflected from moving red blood cells within the lumen is then collected and stored in a computer for subsequent intraluminal image reconstruction.

Echocardiography

Also called heart sonography and sonocardiography, this widely used noninvasive test examines the size, shape, and motion of cardiac structures. Echocardiography helps evaluate patients with abnormal heart sounds, chest pain, electrocardiographic changes unrelated to coronary artery disease, and an enlarged heart seen on X-ray. The test also examines left ventricular function and detects some complications after myocardial infarction (MI).

To perform the procedure, an examiner places a special transducer at an acoustic window (an area where bones and lung tissue are absent) on the patient's chest. He may, for example, place the transducer at the third or fourth intercostal space just to the left of the sternum. The transducer then directs ultrahigh-frequency sound waves toward cardiac structures and picks up the echoes (or reflected waves). These echoes are converted to electrical impulses and relayed to an echocardiography machine for display on an oscilloscope screen and recording on a strip chart or videotape. Electrocardiography and phonocardiography may be performed simultaneously to time events in the cardiac cycle.

The two most common echocardiography techniques are M-mode echocardiography and two-dimensional echocardiography. In *M-mode echocardiography,* a single columnar ultrasonic beam strikes the heart, producing a vertical view of cardiac structures. This technique is especially useful for precisely recording the motion and dimensions of intracardiac structures. In *two-dimensional echocardiography,* the ultrasonic beam rapidly sweeps through an arc, producing a cross-sectional or fan-shaped view of cardiac structures. This technique is useful for recording lateral motion and providing the correct spatial relationships among cardiac structures. In many cases, these two techniques complement each other.

(See *Comparing M-mode and two-dimensional echocardiography.*)

Purpose
● To diagnose and evaluate valvular abnormalities
● To measure the size of the heart chambers
● To evaluate the heart chambers and valves in a patient with a congenital heart disorder
● To aid in diagnosing hypertrophic and related cardiomyopathies
● To detect atrial tumors
● To evaluate cardiac function or wall motion after an MI
● To detect pericardial effusion.

Procedure-related nursing care
Besides performing the nursing care discussed in the chapter introduction, take the following specific measures. Inform the patient that he may be asked to breathe in and out slowly, to hold his breath, or to inhale a gas with a slightly sweet odor (amyl nitrite) while changes in heart function are recorded. Describe the possible adverse effects of amyl nitrite (dizziness, flushing, and tachycardia), but assure him that such symptoms subside quickly.

Normal results
Echocardiography should reveal normal heart size and position as well as normal motion pattern and structure of the four heart valves and the chamber walls.

Abnormal results
Echocardiogram abnormalities may point to various cardiac disorders, such as mitral stenosis, mitral valve prolapse, aortic insufficiency, aortic or subaortic stenosis, tricuspid valve disease, atrial tumors, pericardial effusion, congenital heart disease, an enlarged heart chamber, pulmonary valve insufficiency, cardiac

Comparing M-mode and two-dimensional echocardiography

In the illlustration below, the two shaded areas beneath the transducer indicate the different views of the heart obtained by M-mode and two-dimensional echocardiography. In M-mode echocardiography, the area is columnar (shown in purple), and echo tracings are plotted against time. In two-dimensional echocardiography, the scanning area comprises an arc of 30 degrees (shown in gray), and the scan shows a continuous display.

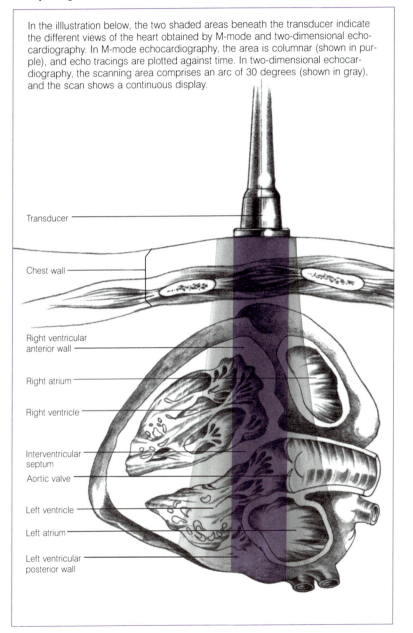

Transducer

Chest wall

Right ventricular anterior wall

Right atrium

Right ventricle

Interventricular septum

Aortic valve

Left ventricle

Left atrium

Left ventricular posterior wall

tamponade, ventricular aneurysm, and cardiomyopathies. For a definitive diagnosis, echocardiogram results should be correlated with the patient's health history and physical examination findings, as well as with the results of other diagnostic studies.

Nursing implications of abnormal results

If the echocardiogram findings confirm valvular heart disease, focus on maintaining adequate cardiac output, controlling pain, preventing complications (such as arrhythmias, infection, and congestive heart failure), and teaching the patient about the need for follow-up assessment, preventive care measures, and possible surgical repair.

If the findings indicate a congenital heart defect, help the infant's parents to understand and accept the condition and teach them precautions to help prevent complications. When indicated, prepare the child and the parents for surgical intervention.

If the findings reveal poor left ventricular function, focus on maintaining cardiac output, preventing congestive heart failure, and teaching the patient about follow-up care, medical treatment, and possible surgical intervention.

If the findings confirm pericardial effusion, monitor the patient for signs of cardiac compression and explain the plan of care.

Gallbladder and biliary system ultrasonography

In ultrasonography of the gallbladder and the biliary system, a focused beam of high-frequency sound waves passes into the right upper abdominal quadrant, creating echoes that vary with changes in tissue density. After these echoes are converted to electrical energy and amplified by the transducer, they appear on an oscilloscope screen as a pattern of spikes or dots. This pattern reveals the size, shape, and position of the gallbladder and may outline a portion of the biliary system.

Because the accuracy of this test doesn't depend on hepatic and gallbladder function, it's especially useful for evaluating patients with elevated serum bilirubin levels when contrast radiography proves ineffective. Ultrasonography also is the procedure of choice for distinguishing between obstructive and nonobstructive jaundice and for making an emergency diagnosis when a patient has symptoms of acute cholecystitis, such as right upper quadrant pain, either with or without local tenderness.

Purpose
- To confirm a diagnosis of cholelithiasis
- To diagnose acute cholecystitis
- To distinguish between obstructive and nonobstructive jaundice.

Procedure-related nursing care

Besides performing the nursing care discussed in the chapter introduction, take the following specific measures. Explain to the patient that he'll be asked to hold his breath periodically and to change positions during the procedure. The evening before the procedure, provide a fat-free meal and withhold food and fluids for 8 to 12 hours. This promotes bile accumulation in the gallbladder and enhances ultrasound visualization.

Normal results

Ultrasonography should reveal normal size, contour, and position of the gallbladder, cystic duct, and common bile duct.

Abnormal results

Abnormal ultrasonographic findings may point to cholelithiasis, cholecystitis, polyps within the gallbladder, or a gallbladder tumor.

Nursing implications of abnormal results

If the test shows biliary tract disease, discuss surgical intervention with the patient, as indicated.

Liver ultrasonography

This ultrasonographic examination produces cross-sectional images of the liver, using high-frequency sound waves directed into the right upper abdominal quadrant. The resulting echoes are converted to electrical energy that appears as a pattern of spikes or dots on an oscilloscope screen. Because this pattern varies with tissue density, it can depict intrahepatic structures as well as liver size, shape, and position.

Liver ultrasonography is indicated for patients who have jaundice of unknown etiology, unexplained hepatomegaly and abnormal biochemical test results, or suspected metastatic tumors and elevated serum alkaline phosphatase levels.

Purpose

• To distinguish between obstructive and nonobstructive jaundice
• To screen for hepatocellular disease
• To detect hepatic metastases and hematoma

• To define tumors, abscesses, or cysts.

Procedure-related nursing care

Besides performing the nursing care discussed in the chapter introduction, take the following specific measures. Explain to the patient that during each scan, he'll be asked to hold his breath briefly after a deep inspiration. Be sure to withhold food and fluids for 8 to 12 hours before the procedure to reduce bowel gas, which impairs ultrasonic wave transmission.

Normal results

Ultrasonography should reveal normal liver size, shape, and position.

Abnormal results

Abnormal ultrasonographic findings may indicate biliary duct obstruction, metastatic liver cancer, primary hepatic tumors, or intrahepatic abscesses, cysts, or hematomas.

Nursing implications of abnormal results

If ultrasonography fails to provide a definitive diagnosis, prepare the patient for such additional tests as a computed tomography scan, gallium scanning, or liver biopsy.

Pancreatic ultrasonography

In this noninvasive test, an examiner channels high-frequency sound waves into the epigastric region. The reflected waves are then converted to electrical impulses that produce cross-sectional images of the pancreas on an oscilloscope screen. Because the images vary with tissue density, they represent the size, shape, and position of the pancreas and surrounding viscera.

Although ultrasonography can't provide a sensitive measurement of pancreatic function, it can help detect anatomic abnormalities, such as pancreatic carcinoma and pseudocysts, and can help guide the insertion of biopsy needles.

Purpose
• To aid in diagnosing pancreatitis, pseudocysts, and pancreatic carcinoma
• To aid biopsy needle insertion.

Procedure-related nursing care
Besides performing the nursing care discussed in the chapter introduction, take the following specific measures. Inform the patient that the examiner will have him lie supine and ask him to inhale deeply and remain as still as possible during the procedure to help ensure accurate results.

Instruct the patient to avoid food and fluids for 8 to 12 hours before the test to reduce bowel gas, which hinders ultrasonic wave transmission. If the patient smokes, ask him to abstain before the test. This eliminates the chance of swallowing air while inhaling; swallowed air interferes with accurate findings.

Normal results
Ultrasonography should reveal a normal-sized pancreas in the proper position.

Abnormal results
Abnormal ultrasonographic findings may point to pancreatitis, pancreatic carcinoma, or pseudocysts.

Nursing implications of abnormal results
As ordered, prepare the patient for more definitive testing — such as a computed tomography scan and biopsy of the pancreas — to diagnose any abnormalities revealed by ultrasonography.

Pelvic ultrasonography

In this test, a piezoelectric crystal generates high-frequency sound waves that are directed at the pelvic area. When the waves are reflected to the transducer, they're converted into electrical energy, forming images of the interior pelvic area on an oscilloscope screen. The most common uses of pelvic ultrasonography include evaluating pelvic disease, assessing fetal growth during pregnancy, and determining fetal

Vaginal probe ultrasonography

In this procedure, sound waves are transmitted to an oscilloscope screen by a probe that the patient inserts into her vagina. Used to assess fetal location and viability in early pregnancy, the test can be used as soon as 5½ weeks after conception. This form of ultrasonography also may be used to evaluate various gynecologic disorders, particularly in obese women.

Procedure-related nursing care
Explain the test's purpose to the patient and describe the procedure. Reassure her that the probe is clean and won't cause discomfort. Tell her the probe will be covered with a lubricated condom before she inserts it.

position before amniocentesis. (Also see *Vaginal probe ultrasonography*.)

Purpose

- To detect foreign bodies, such as intrauterine devices
- To distinguish between cystic and solid masses (tumors)
- To measure organ size
- To diagnose ectopic pregnancy
- To evaluate fetal viability, position, gestational age, and growth rate and to assess the quantity of amniotic fluid
- To guide amniocentesis or chorionic villi sampling by determining the location of the placenta and the position of the fetus
- To detect a multiple pregnancy
- To confirm fetal abnormalities (such as molar pregnancy and abnormalities of the arms and legs, spine, heart, head, kidneys, and abdomen) and maternal abnormalities (such as posterior placenta and placenta previa).

Procedure-related nursing care

Besides performing the nursing care discussed in the chapter introduction, take the following specific measures. Instruct the patient to avoid gas-producing foods, such as carbonated beverages and beans, for 1 to 2 days before the test. Have her drink 32 oz of water or another liquid before the procedure and avoid urinating until the procedure is over; a full bladder provides a useful landmark for identifying pelvic organs. (Also see *Managing supine hypotension*.)

After the test, allow the patient to void.

Normal results

Ultrasonography should reveal a uterus of normal size and shape and ovaries of normal size, shape, and sonographic density, with no other

Managing supine hypotension

During pelvic ultrasonography, a pregnant woman may develop supine hypotension and experience nausea, vertigo, and light-headedness. These complications result from the pressure of the uterus on the abdominal aorta and the inferior vena cava. To relieve these problems, the examiner can turn the patient to the lateral recumbent position.

visible masses. For a pregnant patient, the gestational sac and fetus should be of normal size, the amount of amniotic fluid within normal limits for gestational age, and the placenta properly located. Ultrasonography can reveal a multiple pregnancy after 13 to 14 weeks gestation.

Abnormal results

Pelvic ultrasonography may reveal oligohydramnios, polyhydramnios, a cystic mass, a solid mass, a foreign body, placenta previa, or abruptio placentae. The procedure may also reveal fetal abnormalities, fetal malpresentation, cephalopelvic disproportion, inappropriate fetal size for gestational age, or a dead fetus.

Nursing implications of abnormal results

Provide emotional support to the patient and her family if test results indicate an abnormality, such as a cyst, tumor, or fetal problem. Make sure you understand the prescribed care plan so you can reinforce the doctor's explanations and provide informed answers to any questions the patient and family members may ask.

Renal ultrasonography

In this test, high-frequency sound waves are transmitted from a transducer at the kidneys and perirenal structures. The resulting echoes, amplified and converted into electrical impulses, are displayed on an oscilloscope screen as anatomic images.

Usually performed in conjunction with other urologic tests, renal ultrasonography can detect abnormalities or clarify those revealed by other tests. A safe, painless procedure, it's especially valuable when excretory urography has been ruled out — for example, because of patient hypersensitivity to the contrast medium or because of the need for serial examinations. Unlike excretory urography, this test doesn't depend on renal function and thus can be useful in patients with renal failure.

Purpose
• To determine the size, shape, and position of the kidneys, their internal structures, and perirenal tissues
• To evaluate and locate a urinary tract obstruction and abnormal fluid accumulation
• To assess and diagnose complications after kidney transplantation.

Procedure-related nursing care
Besides performing the nursing care discussed in the chapter introduction, inform the patient that he may be asked to take some deep breaths during the procedure to allow an assessment of kidney movement during respirations.

Normal results
Ultrasonography should reveal kidneys of normal size, shape, and position.

Abnormal results
The test may reveal renal cysts, tumors, or abscesses and adrenal cysts or tumors. Findings also can signal such problems as advanced pyelonephritis or glomerulonephritis, hydronephrosis, ureteral obstruction, congenital anomalies, renal hypertrophy, and rejection of a transplanted kidney.

Nursing implications of abnormal results
If the results indicate a renal disorder, provide emotional support to the patient and his family. Make sure you understand the treatment plan so you can reinforce the doctor's explanations, answer questions accurately, and develop an appropriate care plan. If indicated, prepare the patient for additional diagnostic studies.

Thyroid ultrasonography

In this safe, noninvasive procedure, ultrasonic pulses are directed at the thyroid gland. The reflected pulses are then converted electronically to produce a structural image on an oscilloscope screen.

The test can be used to differentiate between a cyst and a tumor larger than $\frac{1}{8}''$ (0.32 cm) with about 85% accuracy. Because thyroid ultrasonography doesn't expose a fetus to the radioactive iodine used in other diagnostic procedures, the test is particularly useful for evaluating thyroid nodules in pregnant patients.

Ultrasound examination of the parathyroid glands involves much the same procedure as the thyroid study (see *Parathyroid ultrasonography*).

Purpose
- To evaluate thyroid structure and size
- To differentiate between a cyst and a tumor
- To determine the depth and dimension of thyroid nodules.

Procedure-related nursing care
Perform the general nursing care discussed in the chapter introduction.

Normal results
Ultrasonography should reveal a thyroid of normal size and shape.

Abnormal results
Thyroid ultrasonography may reveal cysts, tumors, or nodules.

Nursing implications of abnormal results
If the test results indicate a thyroid cyst, tumor, or nodule, support the patient emotionally and prepare him for any scheduled tests, such as needle biopsy and radionuclide scanning.

   If ultrasonography was performed to monitor thyroid gland size in a patient with a previously diagnosed goiter and the results don't show an appropriate decrease in size, expect the doctor to order a change in the medication regimen.

Urinary bladder ultrasonography

In this procedure, the examiner first places the ultrasound transducer on the patient's abdominal wall over a full bladder to produce an image of the bladder and adjacent structures. Then, after the patient voids, the

Parathyroid ultrasonography

> On ultrasonography, the parathyroid glands appear as solid masses, 5 mm or smaller, with an echo pattern of lower amplitude than that produced by thyroid tissue. If the patient has a tumor growth or hyperplasia, the parathyroid glands will appear larger than 5 mm.

examiner repeats the procedure to determine if any residual urine remains in the bladder. If any does, its volume can be calculated.

Purpose
- To detect residual urine
- To detect structural changes in the bladder wall
- To detect an overdistended bladder
- To detect a bladder tumor and to determine the extent of tumor invasion.

Procedure-related nursing care
Besides performing the nursing care discussed in the chapter introduction, take the following specific measures. Explain to the patient that he'll be examined first with his bladder full and then again after he voids. Tell him that he'll experience some discomfort from bladder distention. But reassure him that the examiner will try to minimize the duration of this discomfort. Instruct the patient to drink several glasses of fluid beginning a few hours before the procedure and to avoid urinating. Explain that a full bladder is necessary to ensure accurate findings.

Normal results
Ultrasonography should reveal a bladder of normal size and contour,

with no significant residual urine and no masses within or outside the bladder wall.

Abnormal results

Ultrasonography may identify an abnormally distended bladder, residual urine, bladder tumors, and masses or fluid accumulation outside the bladder. It may also reveal bladder calculi, cystitis, bladder diverticula, and ureteroceles.

Nursing implications of abnormal results

If findings indicate a bladder disorder, explain the care plan to the patient. Also prepare him for additional diagnostic tests as indicated.

Suggested readings

Diagnostics, 2nd ed. Nurse's Reference Library. Springhouse, Pa.: Springhouse Corp., 1987.

Diagnostic Tests. Nurse's Ready Reference. Springhouse, Pa.: Springhouse Corp., 1991.

Fischbach, F.T. *A Manual of Laboratory Diagnostic Tests,* 3rd ed. Philadelphia: J.B. Lippincott Co., 1988.

Kee, J.L. *Handbook of Laboratory and Diagnostic Tests with Nursing Implications.* Norwalk, Conn.: Appleton & Lange, 1990.

Speicher, C.E. *The Right Test: A Physician's Guide to Laboratory Medicine.* Philadelphia: W.B. Saunders Co., 1989.

7

ENDOSCOPY

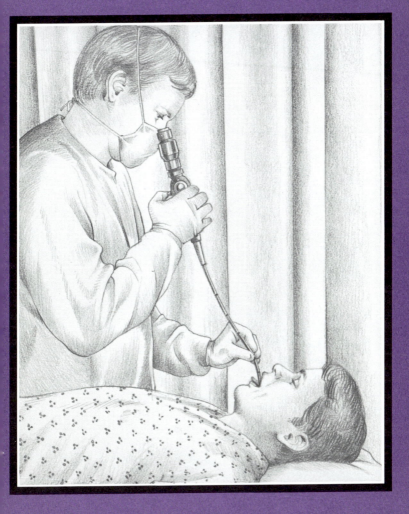

In endoscopic studies, a doctor inserts a rigid or flexible endoscope into a body viscus or joint so he can view internal structures and, sometimes, perform procedures that may eliminate the need for open surgery. Endoscopy can be used to view several areas of the body, including the tracheobronchial tree, the GI tract, and certain joints.

The endoscope itself comes with several features. For instance, valves on the eyepiece allow the use of light, air, or water during the study. Plus, the endoscope can be attached to suction equipment. The device also has channels to accommodate biopsy forceps, a cytology brush, snares, and other equipment, allowing the examiner to perform minor surgery, such as removal of polyps or foreign bodies or cautery of a bleeding point. He also may be able to use a camera. One type of endoscope, the video endoscope, can transmit images to a monitor.

Rigid endoscopes, such as the proctoscope, have a larger internal diameter than flexible endoscopes. Thus, a doctor can remove larger specimens as well as secretions or excretions blocking his view. Unlike the flexible instruments, however, rigid endoscopes can be inserted only for short, straight distances.

Slim, flexible endoscopes allow the doctor to view distant structures (such as the bronchial tree and colon) and out-of-the-way structures (such as the larynx and the nasopharynx). In contrast to rigid endoscopes, these devices generally produce only minor discomfort.

An endoscopic procedure may be performed at the bedside or in a treatment room, an operating room, or the radiology department.

Procedure-related nursing care
The following nursing care measures apply to all endoscopic procedures covered in this chapter. As part of the discussion of each procedure, you'll also find specific nursing care considerations.

Before the procedure. Begin preparing a patient for endoscopy by describing the procedure and explaining its purpose. Describe the equipment, any sensations or discomfort he can expect, and the positions he'll be asked to assume. Your explanations should help reduce any anxiety associated with the unfamiliar and unexpected.

Tell the patient he'll probably be given a sedative. For most endoscopic studies, an antianxiety agent, such as diazepam (Valium), will be given immediately before the procedure to alleviate anxiety and promote relaxation. Explain that he also may receive an analgesic, such as meperidine (Demerol), either just before or during the procedure. Inform the patient that these medications may cause drowsiness and that he may sleep during the procedure. Advise an outpatient to arrange for transportation home, explaining that he shouldn't drive for about 12 hours after receiving a sedative.

If a local anesthetic will be used, explain to the patient that it'll help ease his discomfort during the procedure but that it won't affect his level of consciousness. If general anesthesia is indicated, explain to the patient or to the parents (if the patient is a young child) that he won't be conscious during the procedure. For a patient receiving a general anesthetic, provide standard preoperative nursing care.

Before endoscopy, check the patient's record for a recent barium study. Whenever possible, endoscopy should precede a barium study because residual barium can interfere with accurate findings.

Next, prepare the patient physically for the type of endoscopy he'll undergo. For example, before colonoscopy, the large intestine must be thoroughly cleansed. In this case, follow the prescribed dietary, laxative, enema, or lavage regimen.

After the doctor has explained the procedure and its possible risks, make sure the patient (or guardian) has signed an informed consent form.

During the procedure. If you're present during the procedure, you'll assist the doctor as necessary. Ensure that any equipment to be used, such as a cardiac monitor or an oximeter, is functioning properly. You'll also monitor the patient's vital signs and watch for adverse drug reactions. You may be responsible for sending the specimen to the laboratory for analysis.

After the procedure. Provide care, such as monitoring vital signs, until the patient's condition stabilizes.

Tissue trauma from endoscope insertion can cause complications after the procedure. So assess the patient carefully for signs and symptoms of perforation and bleeding. If you note such findings, notify the doctor and intervene appropriately. Also, continue to monitor the patient for adverse drug reactions.

Provide an outpatient with written instructions on postprocedure care, if indicated.

Arthroscopy

A visual examination of a joint with a specially designed fiber-optic endoscope, arthroscopy is most com-

monly used to assess the knee. Other applications include the shoulder and ankle. (See *Arthroscopy of the knee,* page 158.)

For evaluating a patient with suspected or confirmed joint disease, arthroscopy usually is considered a secondary tool. The initial diagnostic approach consists of a complete history and physical examination plus X-rays and arthrography. However, the diagnostic accuracy of arthroscopy (about 98%) surpasses that of X-rays and arthrography. Thus, arthroscopy may prove to be the definitive diagnostic procedure.

Unlike radiographic studies, arthroscopy permits concurrent surgery or tissue biopsy using a technique known as triangulation, in which instruments are passed through a separate cannula. Thus, arthroscopy provides a safe, convenient alternative to open surgery (arthrotomy) or a separate biopsy. Although arthroscopy is commonly performed using a local anesthetic, it may be done using a spinal or general anesthetic, particularly when complex surgery is anticipated. Arthroscopy is contraindicated when the patient has a wound or a severe skin infection.

Purpose
- To detect and diagnose meniscal, patellar, condylar, extrasynovial, and synovial diseases
- To monitor the progression of disease
- To perform joint surgery.

Procedure-related nursing care
Besides performing the nursing care discussed in the chapter introduction, take the following specific measures.

Before the procedure. Explain to the patient that the procedure allows di-

Arthroscopy of the knee

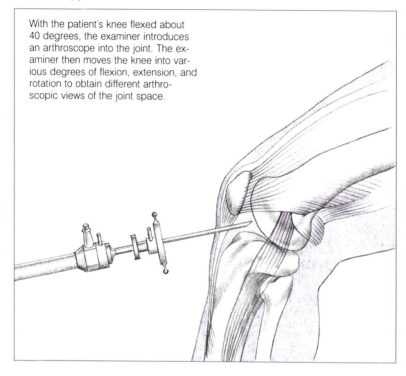

With the patient's knee flexed about 40 degrees, the examiner introduces an arthroscope into the joint. The examiner then moves the knee into various degrees of flexion, extension, and rotation to obtain different arthroscopic views of the joint space.

rect examination of the inside of the joint and is a safe, convenient approach for surgery. Tell him that the procedure will be done in the operating room, using a local, spinal, or general anesthetic, and will involve creating a small incision in the skin over the joint and inserting an arthroscope into the joint cavity. If a local anesthetic will be used, tell the patient that he may feel transient discomfort during the injection.

Withhold food and fluids after midnight the night before the test. Check the patient's record for a history of hypersensitivity to the prescribed anesthetic agent, and report any hypersensitivity to the doctor. Also assess the patient for and re-

port any local skin or wound infections.

Shave and clean an area 5″ (13 cm) above and below the joint; administer the prescribed preprocedure medications; insert an I.V. line, as ordered; and take baseline vital signs.

After the procedure. Administer an analgesic and apply ice to the joint, as ordered. Inform the patient that he may walk as soon as he's fully awake but should avoid excessive joint use for several days. Allow him to resume his normal diet. Explain that he'll probably feel mild soreness and a slight grinding sensation in his joint for 1 or 2 days.

Instruct him to notify the doctor of severe or increased pain or any signs of infection, such as fever and local inflammation.

Reinforce the doctor's instructions concerning exercise, ice application, and dressing changes. Also monitor the patient for complications, such as infection, hemarthrosis (blood accumulation in the joint), and synovial cyst.

Normal results
Normal arthroscopy findings include a joint surrounded by muscles, ligaments, cartilage, and tendons and lined with synovial membrane.

Abnormal results
Arthroscopy may reveal such abnormalities as subluxation, fracture, degenerative articular cartilage, osteochondritis, loose bodies from osteochondral and chondral fractures, torn ligaments, Baker's cyst, ganglionic cyst, synovitis, rheumatoid and degenerative arthritis, and foreign bodies associated with gout. Knee arthroscopy can also detect meniscal injury, chondromalacia patellae, and patellar dislocation.

Nursing implications of abnormal results
Reinforce the doctor's explanations and answer the patient's questions. If the findings indicate the need for major surgery, prepare the patient for the scheduled procedure and provide emotional support.

If the findings reveal a joint disorder, intervene as appropriate to make the patient comfortable. Teach the patient about his prescribed medications, physical therapy, and activity restrictions, such as limitations on weight bearing for a knee disorder. Encourage him to participate in the prescribed physical therapy program.

Bronchoscopy

This diagnostic procedure allows a direct visual examination of the tracheobronchial tree through a standard metal bronchoscope or a flexible fiber-optic bronchoscope. The most commonly used device, the flexible fiber-optic bronchoscope allows a greater view of the segmental and subsegmental bronchi and carries less risk of trauma than the rigid bronchoscope. (See *How a flexible bronchoscope works,* page 160.) However, a large rigid bronchoscope is needed to remove foreign objects, excise endobronchial lesions, and control massive hemoptysis.

Purpose
● To examine a possible tumor, obstruction, secretion, or foreign body in the tracheobronchial tree, as demonstrated on radiography
● To help diagnose bronchogenic carcinoma, tuberculosis, interstitial pulmonary disease, or fungal or parasitic pulmonary infection by obtaining a specimen for bacteriologic and cytologic examination
● To locate a bleeding site in the tracheobronchial tree
● To remove foreign bodies and tumors
● To suction secretions or mucus plugs from the small airways.

Procedure-related nursing care
Besides performing the nursing care discussed in the chapter introduction, take the following specific measures.

Before the procedure. Tell the patient that he'll be placed supine on a table or bed, or asked to sit upright

How a flexible bronchoscope works

Inserted through the patient's nostril and into the bronchi, the flexible fiber-optic bronchoscope has four channels (see enlargement). Two light channels (A) provide a light source; one visualizing channel (B) allows direct examination; and one open channel (C) can accommodate biopsy forceps, a cytology brush, an anesthetic, or oxygen, as well as suctioning or lavage.

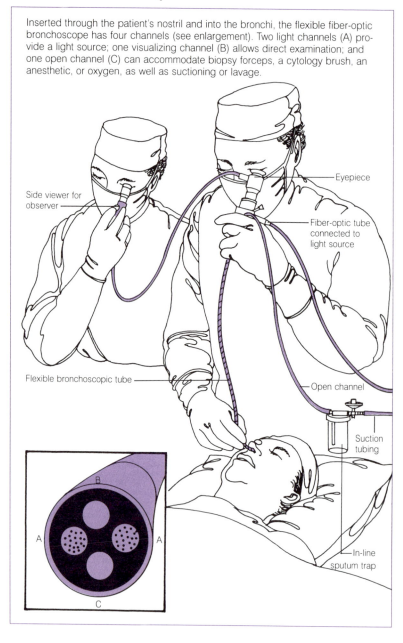

Side viewer for observer

Eyepiece

Fiber-optic tube connected to light source

Flexible bronchoscopic tube

Open channel

Suction tubing

In-line sputum trap

in a chair. Explain that the doctor will introduce the bronchoscope through the nose or mouth and into the airway. He'll then flush small amounts of anesthetic through the tube to suppress coughing and wheezing. Reassure the patient that although he may experience mild discomfort and dyspnea during the procedure, he won't suffocate. Explain that oxygen will be administered through the bronchoscope.

Withhold food and fluids for 6 to 12 hours before the procedure. Tell the patient food, fluids, and oral drugs will be withheld for about 2 hours after the procedure until his gag reflex returns. Then he can have sips of clear liquid or ice chips.

Tell the patient that a chest X-ray may be taken and he may receive an aerosolized bronchodilator treatment after bronchoscopy. Reassure him that any postprocedure hoarseness, loss of voice, or throat soreness will be only temporary and that he can have throat lozenges or gargle as soon as his gag reflex returns.

Check the patient's record for any history of hypersensitivity to the drugs that may be used during the procedure. Obtain baseline vital signs and begin an I.V. infusion, as ordered. Then administer the prescribed preoperative sedatives and analgesics. If the patient is wearing dentures, have him remove them just before the procedure.

During the procedure. If you assist with the procedure, help the patient into the proper position. Tell him to remain relaxed with his arms at his sides throughout the procedure. Monitor him for signs of an adverse reaction to the sedative. Send any specimens to the laboratory at once.

After the procedure. Monitor the patient's vital signs, breath sounds,

and gag reflex. Perform routine postoperative interventions according to hospital policy. As ordered, place a conscious patient in semi-Fowler's position. Place an unconscious patient on his side with the head of the bed slightly elevated.

Provide an emesis basin, and instruct a conscious patient to spit out saliva rather than swallow it. Inspect the sputum for blood, and notify the doctor immediately if excessive bleeding occurs. If ordered, collect all sputum for 24 hours for cytologic examination. Irritation caused by bronchial brushing commonly results in delayed shedding of malignant cells.

Instruct a patient who had a biopsy to refrain from clearing his throat and coughing. Explain that this could dislodge the clot at the biopsy site and cause bleeding.

Assess the patient for signs of complications (see *Managing postbronchoscopy problems,* page 162). Keep resuscitation equipment and a tracheostomy tray readily available for 24 hours after the procedure.

Normal results
Normally, the trachea, a 4½" (11.4-cm) tube extending from the larynx to the mainstem bronchi, consists of smooth muscle containing C-shaped rings of cartilage at regular intervals. This tube is lined with ciliated mucosa. The bronchi appear structurally similar to the trachea. The right mainstem bronchus is slightly shorter, wider, and more vertical than the left mainstem bronchus. Smaller secondary bronchi, bronchioles, alveolar ducts, and eventually alveolar sacs and alveoli branch off the mainstem bronchi.

Abnormal results
Bronchoscopy may reveal various abnormalities of the bronchial wall,

Managing postbronchoscopy problems

SIGNS AND SYMPTOMS	COMPLICATION	NURSING INTERVENTIONS
Subcutaneous crepitus around patient's face and neck	Tracheal or bronchial perforation	• Notify doctor immediately. • Prepare patient for emergency surgery or chest tube insertion.
Laryngeal stridor, dyspnea	Laryngeal edema or laryngospasm	• Notify doctor immediately. • Administer bronchodilators or cool aerosol treatment, as ordered. • Prepare for a possible tracheotomy.
Wheezing, dyspnea	Bronchospasm	• Notify doctor immediately. • Administer oxygen and bronchodilators, as ordered.
Decreased or absent breath sounds on one side; sharp, pleuritic chest pain; dyspnea; cyanosis	Pneumothorax	• Notify doctor immediately. • Place patient in sitting position. • Administer oxygen, as ordered. • Prepare for chest tube insertion.
Excessive hemoptysis	Bleeding or hemorrhage from respiratory tract, especially from biopsy site	• Notify doctor immediately. • Monitor vital signs. • Initiate I.V. therapy, as ordered. • Maintain airway patency. • Prepare patient for a return to surgery.

including inflammation, swelling, protruding cartilage, ulceration, tumors, and enlargement of the mucous gland orifices or submucosal lymph nodes; abnormalities of endotracheal origin, including stenosis, compression, ectasia (dilation of tubular vessels), anomalous (irregular) bronchial branching, and abnormal bifurcation due to a diverticulum; and abnormal substances in the bronchial lumen, such as blood, secretions, calculi, or foreign bodies.

The results of tissue and cell studies may indicate interstitial pulmonary disease, bronchogenic carcinoma, and tuberculosis or other pulmonary infections. A definitive diagnosis requires correlating bronchoscopic findings with radiographic and cytologic findings as well as with clinical signs and symptoms.

Nursing implications of abnormal results
If the results indicate the need for major surgery, prepare the patient as appropriate. If a respiratory disorder is diagnosed, provide support for the patient and reinforce the

doctor's explanations of the disorder and the treatment plan. Initiate measures to promote comfort and provide maximum ventilation.

If bronchoscopy was performed to remove secretions or mucus plugs, perform chest physiotherapy and encourage fluid intake, as ordered, to help clear secretions.

Colonoscopy

When a patient has a history of chronic constipation or diarrhea, persistent rectal bleeding, or lower abdominal pain, and the results of proctosigmoidoscopy and barium enema prove negative or inconclusive, a doctor will perform colonoscopy. In most cases, histologic and cytologic examinations of the specimens obtained will confirm a diagnosis.

To perform this examination of the lining of the large intestine, the doctor may use either a flexible fiber-optic or video colonoscope. Generally a safe procedure, colonoscopy can produce complications, such as perforation of the large intestine, excessive bleeding, and retroperitoneal emphysema.

Purpose
• To perform diagnostic and therapeutic procedures, such as biopsy, cultures, cytologic tests, polypectomy, electrocoagulation, foreign body removal, and stricture dilatation
• To detect or evaluate inflammatory and ulcerative bowel disease
• To locate the origin of lower GI bleeding
• To aid in diagnosing colonic strictures and benign or malignant lesions

• To evaluate the colon postoperatively for recurrence of polyps or malignant lesions.

Procedure-related nursing care
Besides performing the nursing care discussed in the chapter introduction, take the following specific measures.

Before the procedure. Explain that the procedure involves inserting a flexible tube into the anus so the doctor can examine the colon. Inform the patient that he'll lie on an examination table and that he'll receive a sedative and an analgesic.

Assure the patient that the colonoscope will be well lubricated to ease insertion. Explain that he may feel an urge to defecate as the scope is inserted and advanced. Also explain that he may feel cramping or gas pains but that the sedative should help him relax. Tell him to breathe deeply and slowly through his mouth to relax his abdominal muscles during the procedure.

Provide the patient with a clear liquid diet the day before the procedure, then withhold food and fluids starting at midnight on the night before the procedure. To thoroughly clean the large intestine, administer a laxative. For instance, you may give 10 oz (300 ml) of magnesium citrate, 3 tbs (45 ml) of castor oil, or four bisacodyl tablets the evening before the procedure and perform warm tap-water enemas 3 to 4 hours before the test until the return is clear. Don't administer a soapsuds enema because it will irritate the mucosa and stimulate mucus secretions that can hinder the examination. In some institutions, oral lavage solutions, such as Go-LYTELY or Colyte, may be used instead of an enema.

Just before the procedure, start

an I.V. infusion and take the patient's baseline vital signs.

During the procedure. If you assist with the procedure, position the patient on his left side with his knees flexed, and drape him appropriately. As ordered, help the patient to a supine position to ease the advance of the colonoscope when it reaches the descending sigmoid junction.

Monitor the patient for adverse reactions to the sedative, such as respiratory depression, hypotension, excessive diaphoresis, bradycardia, and confusion.

If the doctor removes a tissue specimen, immediately place it in a specimen bottle containing 10% formalin. Immediately place cytology smears in a Copeland jar containing 95% ethyl alcohol. Send the specimens to the laboratory at once.

After the procedure. Assess the patient carefully for signs and symptoms of bowel perforation — malaise, rectal bleeding, abdominal pain and distention, and fever. If you note such signs and symptoms, notify the doctor immediately. Also, monitor the patient's vital signs until they're stable.

Instruct the patient to rest for several hours after the test and to resume a normal diet after he recovers from sedation. Explain that he may pass large amounts of flatus, resulting from the air insufflated to distend the colon. Provide privacy to minimize embarrassment.

Normal results
The mucosa of the large intestine beyond the sigmoid colon appears light pink-orange and is marked by semilunar folds and deep tubular pits. Blood vessels are visible beneath the intestinal mucosa, which glistens from mucus secretions.

Abnormal results
Visual examination of the large intestine, coupled with histologic and cytologic findings, may indicate proctitis, granulomatous or ulcerative colitis, Crohn's disease, or malignant or benign lesions. This examination also may detect diverticular disease or locate the site of lower GI bleeding.

Nursing implications of abnormal results
If the results of colonoscopy indicate the need for major surgery, prepare the patient physically and emotionally. If colonoscopy and biopsy findings point to an intestinal disorder, such as cancer or inflammatory bowel disease, provide emotional support, reinforce the doctor's explanation of the prescribed care plan, and answer any questions the patient has. Refer the patient to support groups, as appropriate.

Cystoscopy

Cystoscopy (or cystourethroscopy) allows direct visual examination of the bladder and urethra, including the prostatic urethra in men. During cystoscopy, the examiner may perform procedures, such as biopsy, dilatation of a constricted urethra, lesion resection, collection of calculi, and retrograde ureteral catheterization. Kidney-ureter-bladder (KUB) radiography and excretory urography usually precede cystoscopy.

Purpose
• To diagnose and evaluate urinary tract disorders.

Procedure-related nursing care
Besides performing the nursing care

discussed in the chapter introduction, take the following specific measures.

Before the procedure. Tell the patient that the doctor will introduce the cystoscope through the urethra into the bladder. Then he'll fill the bladder with irrigating solution and rotate the scope to inspect the entire surface of the bladder wall.

If a general anesthetic will be used, withhold food and fluids for 8 hours before the procedure. If a local anesthetic will be used, tell the patient that he may experience a burning sensation as the instrument passes through the urethra and feel an urgent need to urinate as the bladder is filled with irrigating solution. Reassure him that these sensations are common and usually transient. Also explain that he may experience some discomfort after the procedure, including slight burning on urination.

Check the patient's history for hypersensitivity to drugs that may be used during the test; report any hypersensitivity to the doctor. Just before the procedure, measure and record baseline vital signs, and have the patient urinate. Administer prescribed preprocedure medications.

During the procedure. If you're assisting with the procedure, place the patient in the lithotomy position on the examination table. Collect urine specimens, as ordered. Label all specimens properly and send them to the laboratory immediately.

After the procedure. Instruct the patient to drink fluids freely and to take the prescribed analgesic. Instruct him to abstain from alcohol for 48 hours.

Reassure him that any burning or frequency should subside in 24 to 48 hours. Administer antibiotics, as ordered, to prevent bacterial sepsis from urethral tissue trauma.

Record intake and output for 24 hours, and look for bladder distention. If the patient doesn't void within 8 hours after the test, or if bright red blood continues to appear after three voidings, notify the doctor. Monitor the patient for and immediately report flank or abdominal pain, chills, fever, or oliguria.

Normal results

The urethra, bladder, and ureteral orifices should appear normal in size, shape, and position. The mucosa lining the lower urinary tract should appear smooth and shiny with no evidence of erythema, cysts, or other abnormalities. The bladder should be free of obstructions, tumors, and calculi.

Abnormal results

One of the most common abnormal findings is an enlarged prostate gland in older men. Other common abnormal findings in both men and women include urethral strictures, calculi, tumors or polyps, diverticula, and ulcers. The procedure also may detect bladder wall decompression and various congenital anomalies, such as ureteroceles, duplicated ureteral orifices, or urethral valves.

Nursing implications of abnormal results

If the cystoscopy findings indicate the need for major surgery, prepare the patient physically and emotionally. Also provide physical and emotional support to the patient with a diagnosed bladder disorder. Monitor urine output, and initiate measures to promote effective urine elimination and prevent infection. Reinforce the doctor's explanation of the care required and answer any questions.

Endoscopic retrograde cholangiopancreatography

Endoscopic retrograde cholangiopancreatography (ERCP) uses radiography and endoscopy to examine the pancreatic ducts and the hepatobiliary tree. To perform the procedure, the examiner advances a small, side-viewing endoscope through the mouth, esophagus, and stomach into the duodenum until he can see the ampulla of Vater. Then, after injecting a contrast medium through a catheter in the endoscope, he takes X-rays of the pancreatic and biliary systems. (See *Placing the endoscope for ERCP.*)

ERCP is indicated for patients with confirmed or suspected pancreatic disease and those with obstructive jaundice of unknown origin. With the development of smaller, side-viewing endoscopes, ERCP is becoming a more common procedure.

Purpose
• To evaluate obstructive jaundice
• To help diagnose tumors of the duodenal papilla, the pancreas, and the biliary ducts
• To locate calculi and stenosis in the pancreatic ducts and hepatobiliary tree
• To perform therapeutic procedures, such as papillotomy, calculi removal, stent and drain placement, and biliary dilatation.

Procedure-related nursing care
Besides performing the nursing care discussed in the chapter introduction, take the following specific measures.

Before the procedure. Inform the patient that a local anesthetic may be sprayed into his mouth to suppress his gag reflex and ease insertion of the endoscope. Warn him that the spray has an unpleasant taste and makes the tongue and throat feel swollen, causing swallowing difficulty. Instruct him to let saliva drain from the side of his mouth, and explain that suction may be used if necessary.

Explain that a mouth guard will be inserted to protect the patient's teeth and the endoscope. Assure him that the mouth guard won't obstruct his breathing. A patient with dentures won't need a mouth guard, but explain that he'll have to remove his dentures before the procedure. Also, inform the patient that he may gag as air is pumped into the intestines. Explain that the air helps the examiner view the mucosa.

Tell the patient that he'll receive an I.V. antianxiety agent and analgesic to help him relax. He'll also receive an I.V. anticholinergic or glucagon after the endoscope is inserted. Describe the possible adverse effects of anticholinergics (dry mouth, thirst, tachycardia, urine retention, and blurred vision) or of glucagon (nausea, vomiting, hives, and flushing). Warn him that he may experience transient flushing when the contrast medium is injected and may have a sore throat for about 24 hours after the examination.

Instruct the patient to fast after midnight the night before the procedure. Check his chart for any history of hypersensitivity to seafood, iodine, contrast media used for other diagnostic procedures, or any medications. Also evaluate the results of any laboratory tests; tests commonly ordered before ERCP include a complete blood count, bleeding times, a hepatitis screen, and liver and serum enzyme studies. Be sure to notify the doctor of any hypersensitivity or abnormal test results.

Just before the procedure, obtain and record baseline vital signs. Instruct the patient to remove all metal and other radiopaque objects, and constricting undergarments. Then encourage him to void to minimize the discomfort of urine retention, which may occur if an anticholinergic is administered. If the patient doesn't have a patent I.V. line for drug and fluid infusion,

Placing the endoscope for ERCP

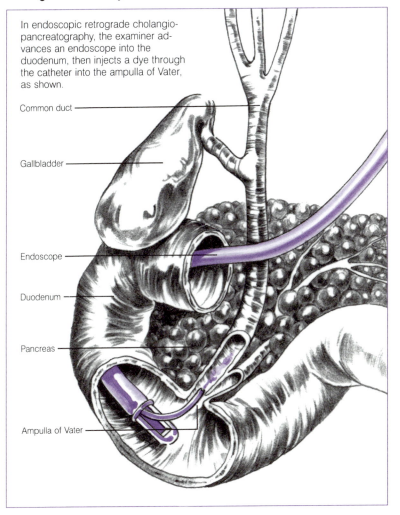

In endoscopic retrograde cholangiopancreatography, the examiner advances an endoscope into the duodenum, then injects a dye through the catheter into the ampulla of Vater, as shown.

Common duct

Gallbladder

Endoscope

Duodenum

Pancreas

Ampulla of Vater

insert one, if ordered. Administer any prescribed preprocedure medications.

During the procedure. If you're assisting with the procedure, make sure that emergency resuscitation equipment and a narcotic antagonist (such as naloxone) are readily available. After the doctor administers the local anesthetic, place the patient in the left lateral position. Instruct him to lie still as the endoscope is inserted and X-rays are taken. When the doctor begins to administer the I.V. medication, monitor the patient for respiratory depression, apnea, hypotension, excessive diaphoresis, bradycardia, and laryngospasm. Assist him to the prone position when instructed to do so. Ensure that all specimens are placed in properly labeled containers and sent to the laboratory immediately.

After the procedure. Help the patient sit up or turn to his side so he can cough and expectorate the thick secretions that accumulated during the test. Make sure you give him extra support as you do this because he'll still be drowsy from the medication. Monitor vital signs until they're stable, comparing them to baseline values. Assess him for signs of urine retention. Notify the doctor if the patient doesn't void within 8 hours.

Watch closely for signs of cholangitis and pancreatitis. Hyperbilirubinemia, fever, and chills are the immediate signs of cholangitis; hypotension associated with gram-negative septicemia may develop later. Left upper quadrant pain and tenderness, elevated serum amylase levels, and transient hyperbilirubinemia are the usual signs of pancreatitis. Draw blood samples for amylase and bilirubin determinations, if ordered, keeping in mind that these levels normally show transient increases after ERCP. (See *Managing ERCP problems.*)

Continue assessing the patient for respiratory depression, apnea, hypotension, excessive diaphoresis, bradycardia, and laryngospasm. Withhold food and fluids until the gag reflex returns, at which time you can allow fluids and a light meal. If the patient complains of a sore throat, provide soothing lozenges and warm saline gargles to ease discomfort.

Normal results

The duodenal papilla appears as a small, red or sometimes pale erosion protruding into the lumen. Its orifice is commonly bordered by a fringe of white mucosa. A longitudinal fold running perpendicular to the deep, circular folds of the duodenum helps mark its location. The pancreatic and hepatobiliary ducts are patent and, although they usually unite in the ampulla of Vater and empty through the duodenal papilla, separate orifices are sometimes present. The contrast medium uniformly fills the pancreatic duct, the hepatobiliary tree, and the gallbladder.

Abnormal results

Examination of the hepatobiliary tree may reveal calculi, strictures, or irregular deviations that suggest biliary cirrhosis, primary sclerosing cholangitis, or bile duct carcinoma. Examination of the pancreatic ducts may also reveal calculi, strictures, or irregular deviations that may indicate pancreatic cysts and pseudocysts, a pancreatic tumor, carcinoma of the head of the pancreas, chronic pancreatitis, pancreatic fibrosis, carcinoma of the duodenal papilla, or papillary stenosis.

Managing ERCP problems

SIGNS AND SYMPTOMS	COMPLICATION	NURSING INTERVENTIONS
• Pain on swallowing and with neck movement • Substernal or epigastric pain that increases with breathing and with movement of trunk • Shoulder pain and dyspnea • Abdominal or back pain, cyanosis, fever, or pleural effusion	Perforation on insertion of endoscope	• Monitor vital signs and provide emotional support. • Assist the doctor as necessary.
• Hyperbilirubinemia, fever, and chills (immediate signs); hypotension associated with gram-negative septicemia (later sign)	Cholangitis	• Monitor vital signs and notify the doctor.
• Left upper quadrant pain and tenderness, elevated serum amylase levels, and transient hyperbilirubinemia	Pancreatitis	• Notify the doctor and anticipate that samples will need to be drawn for serum amylase and bilirubin determinations.

Nursing implications of abnormal results

When the results of ERCP indicate the need for major surgery, prepare the patient physically and emotionally. If the findings suggest a cancer, provide emotional support, reinforce the doctor's explanations of the disorder and care plan, and answer the patient's questions. Do the same for a patient with a diagnosed pancreatic disorder. Also, promote comfort and good nutrition, and watch for signs of insulin deficiency.

Esophagogastro-duodenoscopy

Usually performed by a gastroenterologist, this procedure consists of an endoscopic examination of the esophagus, stomach, and upper duodenum. It also allows the examiner to collect specimens for histologic or cytologic testing if necessary.

Indicated for patients with hematemesis, melena, or substernal or epigastric pain and for postoperative patients with recurrent or new symptoms, esophagogastroduodenoscopy is generally considered safe. However, the procedure can produce perforation of the esophagus, stomach, or duodenum — especially if the patient is restless. For this reason, it's contraindicated for uncooperative patients.

Purpose
• To determine the site and cause of upper GI bleeding
• To diagnose structural abnormalities and upper GI disease
• To obtain a biopsy specimen
• To evaluate the stomach and duo-

denum postoperatively
• To obtain an emergency diagnosis, such as esophageal injury from an ingestion of chemicals.

Procedure-related nursing care
Besides performing the nursing care discussed in the chapter introduction, take the following specific measures.

Before the procedure. Tell the patient that he'll be sedated just before and during the procedure to help him relax. Explain that this will make him feel drowsy. He may also receive an analgesic to help alleviate any discomfort.

Inform the patient that a bitter-tasting local anesthetic may be sprayed into his mouth and throat to suppress the gag reflex. Warn him that this may cause his tongue and throat to feel swollen, making swallowing seem difficult. Advise him to let the saliva drain from the side of his mouth. If necessary, a suction machine may be used to remove saliva.

Instruct the patient to fast for 6 to 12 hours before the test. (For an emergency procedure, the stomach contents may be suctioned to allow a better view.) Explain that a mouth guard will be inserted to protect his teeth and the endoscope. Assure him that the mouth guard won't obstruct his breathing. A patient with dentures won't need a mouth guard, but explain that he'll have to remove his dentures before the procedure.

Tell the patient that he may feel pressure in his stomach as the endoscope is moved about and fullness when air is insufflated. Assure him that he should feel little or no discomfort, however.

Review the patient's record for any history of hypersensitivity to the medications and anesthetic ordered for the test. Report any hypersensitivity to the doctor. Also, check whether the patient has had a recent upper GI series. Esophagogastroduodenoscopy shouldn't be performed within 2 days of an upper GI series because barium retention will hinder the examination.

Check that the patient has a heparin lock or an I.V. site through which medications can be administered. If not, start an I.V. infusion, as ordered. Administer any prescribed preprocedure medications, as ordered. Just before the procedure, instruct the patient to remove eyeglasses, necklaces, hairpins, combs, and constricting undergarments. Measure and record baseline vital signs. Leave the blood pressure cuff in place for monitoring throughout the procedure.

During and after the procedure. If you're assisting with the procedure, you'll have specific responsibilities to carry out (see *Assisting with esophagogastroduodenoscopy*).

After the procedure, monitor vital signs and compare them to baseline values. Also, assess for signs and symptoms of perforation. Perforation in the cervical area of the esophagus produces pain on swallowing and neck movement; thoracic perforation, substernal or epigastric pain that increases with breathing or movement of the trunk; diaphragmatic perforation, shoulder pain and dyspnea; and gastric perforation, abdominal or back pain, cyanosis, fever, and pleural effusion.

Withhold food and fluids until the gag reflex returns. When it does — usually in an hour or so — allow fluids and a light meal, as ordered. Inform the patient that he may burp some insufflated air and may experience a sore throat for about 24

Assisting with esophagogastroduodenoscopy

To assist with the procedure, follow these steps:

● Make sure emergency resuscitation equipment and a narcotic antagonist, such as naloxone, are available.

● Monitor the patient's vital signs throughout the procedure.

● Put on clean gloves, and ask the patient to open his mouth and hold his breath while you spray the anesthetic. Offer him an emesis basin and tissues so he can spit out excess saliva.

● Administer the sedative, as ordered, and be prepared to give more throughout the procedure. (The doctor may administer the medication.)

● Monitor the patient for adverse reactions to the medication: respiratory depression, apnea, hypotension, excessive diaphoresis, bradycardia, and laryngospasm.

● Place the patient in the left lateral position with his head bent forward.

● Ask the patient to open his mouth before the doctor inserts the endoscope, and insert the mouth guard if necessary. Offer emotional support as the endoscope passes through the esophagus, stomach, and duodenum.

● Help the doctor position the patient's head as the endoscope advances. Usually, as the endoscope passes through the posterior pharynx and the cricopharyngeal sphincter, the patient's head is extended and his chin is kept at the midline. When the endoscope reaches the esophagus, the patient's head should be positioned with his chin toward the table, so his saliva can easily drain out of his mouth.

● After the doctor removes the endoscope and mouth guard, wipe the patient's mouth. Help the patient to a comfortable position on his side.

● If tissue specimens have been obtained, place them in a specimen bottle containing 10% formalin solution. Cell specimens should be smeared on glass slides and placed in a Copeland jar containing 95% ethyl alcohol. Label the specimens appropriately, and send them to the laboratory immediately.

hours. Provide throat lozenges and warm saline gargles, as needed. Instruct him to report persistent bleeding, vomiting, pain, abdominal distention, fever, or difficulty swallowing.

Normal results

The smooth esophageal mucosa normally appears yellow-pink and is marked by a fine vascular network. A pulsation on the anterior wall of the esophagus between 8″ and 10″ (20 and 25 cm) from the incisor teeth represents the aortic arch.

The orange-red mucosa of the stomach begins at the Z line, an irregular transition line slightly above the esophagogastric junction. Unlike the esophagus, the stomach has rugal folds, and its blood vessels aren't visible beneath the gastric mucosa.

The reddish mucosa of the duodenal bulb is marked by a few shallow longitudinal folds. In contrast, the distal duodenal mucosa has prominent circular folds, is lined with villi, and appears velvety.

Abnormal results

The visual examination findings, correlated with the results of histologic and cytologic tests, may indicate acute or chronic ulcers, benign or malignant tumors, or inflammatory disease, such as esophagitis, gastritis, or duodenitis. Esophago-gastroduodenoscopy also may detect diverticula, varices, Mallory-Weiss syndrome, esophageal rings, esoph-ageal and pyloric stenoses, or esophageal hiatal hernia. Although esophagogastroduodenoscopy can be used to evaluate gross abnormalities of esophageal motility, such as occur in achalasia, manometric studies generally prove more accurate.

Nursing implications of abnormal results

When the findings indicate the need for major surgery, prepare the pa-tient physically and emotionally. Monitor the patient with an upper GI disorder for signs of blood loss, such as a rapid pulse rate. Also, teach him about the prescribed care plan, reinforcing the doctor's expla-nations and answering any ques-tions. Intervene as appropriate to promote comfort, adequate rest, and optimum nutrition.

Proctosigmoidoscopy

This procedure involves an examina-tion of the lining of the anal canal, rectum, and distal sigmoid colon, sometimes using two different endo-scopes. The doctor uses a sigmoido-scope to examine the anus, rectum, and distal sigmoid colon, and an ano-scope or a proctoscope to examine the anus and rectum. If he uses a flexible sigmoidoscope, he'll also be able to see the descending colon.

Proctosigmoidoscopy is indicated for patients with recent changes in bowel habits, lower abdominal and perineal pain, prolapse on defeca-tion, or anal pruritus as well as for those who've passed mucus, blood,

or pus in their stool. The procedure is also a common component of a routine annual physical examination for persons over age 40.

Purpose
• To aid in diagnosing disorders of the rectosigmoid colon, descending colon, and anal canal.

Procedure-related nursing care

Besides performing the nursing care discussed in the chapter introduc-tion, take the following specific mea-sures.

Before the procedure. Explain to the patient that the doctor will insert a tube into the rectum so he can view the lower GI tract. Inform the pa-tient that he may experience gas pains, abdominal cramping, and the urge to defecate as the tube is in-serted and advanced. Instruct him to breathe deeply and slowly through his mouth during the proce-dure and to relax his abdominal muscles.

Explain to the patient that he may receive an antianxiety agent or a sedative to help him relax and, if or-dered, an analgesic immediately be-fore the procedure to reduce discomfort.

Instruct the patient concerning prescribed dietary restrictions and bowel preparation. If ordered, re-strict food and fluids on the morning of the procedure. Also if ordered, administer a warm tap-water or so-dium biphosphate enema 1 to 2 hours before the procedure.

During and after the procedure. If you're assisting with the procedure, you'll have specific responsibilities to carry out (see *Assisting with proctosigmoidoscopy and anoscopy*).

After the procedure, monitor the patient closely for signs and symp-

Assisting with proctosigmoidoscopy and anoscopy

To assist with these procedures, follow these steps:

• Monitor the patient's vital signs throughout the procedure.

• Place the patient in the left lateral position with his knees flexed or in a knee-to-chest position, as directed by the doctor. When you use the left lateral position, the patient's buttocks should project over the edge of the table. Drape him to minimize embarrassment.

• Tell him to breathe deeply and slowly through his mouth as the doctor performs a digital examination of the anus and rectum.

• Tell the patient when the doctor is ready to insert the sigmoidoscope. Because advancing the scope into the distal sigmoid colon can be uncomfortable, offer the patient encouragement and support. Help the doctor as necessary while he inserts the sigmoidoscope to its full length and then slowly withdraws it.

• To obtain a specimen, the doctor will remove the eyepiece and replace it with a cotton swab used to remove fecal material obstructing vision. The doctor can then insert the biopsy forceps, cytology brush, culture swab, or suction catheter (which removes blood, excessive secretions, or liquid feces) to obtain the specimen. Using an electrocautery snare through the sigmoidoscope, the doctor can also remove polyps.

• After the doctor withdraws the sigmoidoscope, he may need to insert the anoscope. If he does, tell the patient and assure him that it will cause less discomfort than the sigmoidoscope.

• Assist the doctor as he lubricates and inserts the anoscope to its full length and then slowly withdraws it.

• If a specimen is required, the doctor will obtain it as described above. However, if he wants a biopsy of the anal canal, the patient will first need an anesthetic.

• If the procedure was done with the patient in the knee-to-chest position, instruct him to rest in the supine position for several minutes before standing. This will help prevent postural hypotension.

• Either you or the doctor will place the specimens in the appropriate containers. Tissue specimens go in a specimen bottle containing 10% formalin; cytology slides, in a Copeland jar containing 95% ethyl alcohol; and culture swabs, in a culture tube. Label the specimens appropriately, and send them to the laboratory immediately.

toms of bowel perforation (fever, malaise, rectal bleeding, and abdominal distention and pain) and for a vasovagal attack related to emotional stress (decreased blood pressure, pallor, diaphoresis, and bradycardia). Notify the doctor immediately of such findings.

If air was introduced into the intestine, inform the patient that he may pass a large amount of flatus. Provide privacy while he rests after the procedure. If a biopsy or polypectomy was performed, inform him that a small amount of blood may appear in his stool.

Normal results

The mucosa of the sigmoid colon appears light pink-orange with semilunar folds and deep tubular pits. The rectal mucosa appears redder because of its rich vascular network, deepens to a purple hue at the pectinate line (the anatomic division between the rectum and anus), and has three distinct valves. The lower two-thirds of the anus (anoderm) is lined with smooth gray-tan skin and joins with the hair-fringed perianal skin.

Abnormal results

This procedure may detect anorectal abscesses, hemorrhoids, anal fissures, anal fistulas, inflammation or infection, ulcerative colitis, tumors, polyps, strictures, or inflammatory bowel disease.

Nursing implications of abnormal results

If the findings indicate the need for surgery, prepare the patient physically and emotionally. Teach the patient with a rectal or sigmoidal disorder or a diagnosis of cancer about the prescribed care plan. Reinforce the doctor's explanations, and answer the patient's questions.

Suggested readings

Diagnostic Tests. Nurse's Ready Reference. Springhouse, Pa.: Springhouse Corp., 1991.

Fischbach, F.T. *A Manual of Laboratory Diagnostic Tests,* 3rd ed. Philadelphia: J.B. Lippincott Co., 1988.

Kee, J.L. *Handbook of Laboratory and Diagnostic Tests.* Norwalk, Conn.: Appleton & Lange, 1990.

Marta, M.R. "Endoscopic Retrograde Cholangiopancreatography: Its Role in Diagnosis and Treatment," *Focus on Critical Care* 14(5):62-63, October 1987.

Pagana, K.D., and Pagana, T.J. *Diagnostic Testing and Nursing Implications: A Case Study Approach,* 3rd ed. St. Louis: C.V. Mosby Co., 1990.

Speicher, C.E. *The Right Test: A Physician's Guide to Laboratory Medicine.* Philadelphia: W.B. Saunders Co., 1989.

Urban, M.H. "Endoscopic Retrograde Cholangiopancreatography: A Diagnostic Outpatient Procedure," *AORN Journal* 50(3):572-81, September 1989.

8

SPECIAL STUDIES

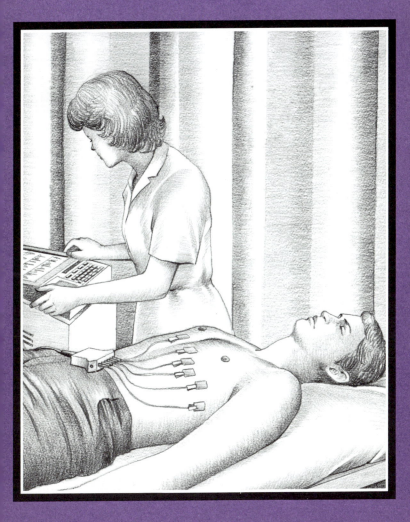

In this final chapter, we'll cover several important diagnostic tests that resist easy classification. They range from complex invasive procedures, such as cardiac catheterization, to fairly simple noninvasive procedures, such as pulmonary function tests.

The invasive procedures, which will be performed by a doctor, present serious risks to the patient. Your primary responsibilities will include preparing the patient for the test and monitoring him for complications afterward. In some cases, you may also assist during the procedure.

You may perform the procedures for some of the noninvasive studies — electrocardiography and pulmonary function tests, for example. Others, such as magnetic resonance imaging, will be performed by a doctor or specially trained technician. But whether you perform the procedure or not, you'll be responsible for preprocedure and postprocedure care.

Procedure-related nursing care

The following nursing care measures apply to all the procedures covered in this chapter. As part of the discussion of each procedure, you'll also find specific nursing care considerations.

Before the procedure. Always explain the purpose of the test to the patient. Describe the procedure, explaining where it will be performed, who will be performing it, and what equipment will be used. Tell the patient if the procedure will cause any discomfort or other sensations.

If he'll receive a local anesthetic, explain that it will alleviate his discomfort but leave him alert. If he'll receive another medication, explain its purpose, the administration route, and any adverse effects.

Help prepare the patient physically for the test, discussing any dietary or activity restrictions. Also, explain any risks the test poses. If the test requires informed consent, check that the patient or a responsible family member has signed the appropriate form.

After the procedure. Perform any special care and enforce necessary restrictions. Be sure to explain to the patient why such care is needed. And monitor him for complications.

Cardiac catheterization

An invasive diagnostic procedure, cardiac catheterization involves inserting a catheter into the right or left side of the heart through a vein or artery of the arm or leg. The examiner uses fluoroscopy to guide catheter insertion and a contrast dye to help see the heart structures. The procedure can be used to help identify, measure, and verify almost every kind of intracardiac problem. (See *Cardiac catheter pathways,* pages 178 and 179.)

Using cardiac catheterization, an examiner can determine blood pressure and blood flow in the heart chambers, collect blood samples, and record films of the ventricles (contrast ventriculography) or arteries (coronary arteriography or angiography). The test also lets the examiner calculate cardiac output.

Catheterization of the right side of the heart permits hemodynamic evaluation of right atrial, right ventricular, and pulmonary artery pressures. The examiner can also assess tricuspid and pulmonary valve function. Catheterization of the left side of the heart allows hemodynamic evaluation of left atrial and left ventricular pressures, as well as mitral and aortic valve function.

Hemodynamic pressures on either side of the heart are measured by an electronic transducer passed through the cardiac catheter. The transducer sends a signal to a monitor, which illustrates the pressure as a waveform. Each cardiac chamber and great vessel has a normal waveform and range of pressure. An elevated pressure in a particular chamber or vessel may indicate a problem.

Hemodynamic measurements also serve as an important diagnostic tool for valvular stenosis. If stenosis is suspected, measurements are taken on each side of the valve. If the valve is stenotic and not functioning properly, blood can't flow normally, creating a pressure buildup. This pressure difference between the two sides of the valve, called a gradient, helps in calculating the area of the valve. When the valve becomes critically narrowed, open-heart valve replacement is usually recommended.

During the hemodynamic portion of the study, blood samples can be taken to evaluate oxygen content.

Besides permitting hemodynamic monitoring, catheterization of the left side of the heart also allows the examiner to view the ventricle and the coronary arteries and to film the heart's activity. The examiner can also assess coronary artery patency and the left ventricular ejection fraction—the percentage of left ventricular blood volume ejected with each ventricular contraction. Using angiography, the examiner can observe the heart's pumping performance, detect coronary artery disease (CAD), and identify vessels that need bypass grafting.

Purpose
• To evaluate valvular insufficiency or stenosis, septal defects, congenital anomalies, myocardial function, coronary circulation, and cardiac wall motion
• To determine if a patient needs coronary artery bypass graft surgery or percutaneous transluminal coronary angioplasty.

Procedure-related nursing care
Besides performing the nursing care discussed in the chapter introduction, take the following specific measures.

Before the procedure. Tell the patient that he'll be strapped to a padded table that can be tilted so his heart can be examined from different angles. Advise him that he may receive a mild sedative but that he'll be conscious during the procedure. Explain that an I.V. needle will be inserted into his arm to deliver medication and that electrodes will be attached to his chest and limbs to monitor his heart rhythm. Be sure to tell him that the electrodes won't cause any discomfort.

Explain that before the catheter is inserted, the insertion site will be shaved and cleaned. Warn the patient that he'll feel a transient stinging sensation when the local anesthetic is injected and that he may feel pressure as the catheter moves through the blood vessel. Explain too that the contrast medium injected through the catheter may produce a transient hot, flushing sensation or nausea. Advise him to cough or breathe deeply, as directed.

During the procedure, the patient may hear a clacking noise as the film advances. Explain that if he develops chest pain, he'll receive medication. He may also be given nitro-

Cardiac catheter pathways

A cardiac catheter can be advanced into either the right or left side of the heart. These illustrations show the most common pathway used to reach each side.

Right side of the heart
This illustration shows the catheter inserted into the femoral vein and advanced through the inferior vena cava, the right atrium, and the right ventricle, and then into the pulmonary artery. As an alternative, the catheter can be inserted into an antecubital vein and advanced through the superior vena cava, the right atrium, and the right ventricle, and then into the pulmonary artery.

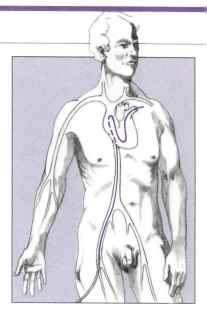

glycerin periodically to dilate his coronary vessels. Reassure him that complications, such as myocardial infarction or thromboemboli, are rare.

Instruct the patient to avoid food and fluids for 4 to 6 hours before the test, as ordered. Also, ask him if he's hypersensitive to shellfish, iodine, or the contrast media used in other diagnostic tests. If so, notify the doctor. Check whether the patient is receiving anticoagulant therapy. If so, notify the doctor immediately; he may decide not to proceed with the cardiac catheterization.

Just before the procedure, tell the patient to void. Take his baseline vital signs and administer any pretest medications, as ordered.

During and after the procedure. If you're present for the procedure, help the patient into the supine position on the cardiac catheterization table. Secure him with the safety belt and apply electrocardiograph (ECG) leads for continuous monitoring. Insert an I.V. line, as ordered.

Provide emotional support during the procedure. A catheterization team will monitor the patient's vital signs.

After the procedure, monitor the patient's vital signs every 15 minutes for the first hour, then every 30 minutes for 2 hours, and then every hour for 4 hours to make sure he remains stable. If his condition isn't stable, check his vital signs every 5 minutes and notify the doctor.

Observe the catheter insertion site for a hematoma or bleeding — both serious complications (see *Managing cardiac catheterization problems,* pages 180 to 182). To prevent hematoma formation and

Left side of the heart

This illustration shows the catheter inserted into the femoral artery and advanced through the aorta and the aortic valve, and then into the left ventricle. As an alternative, the catheter can be inserted into the brachial artery and advanced through the aorta and the aortic valve, and then into the left ventricle.

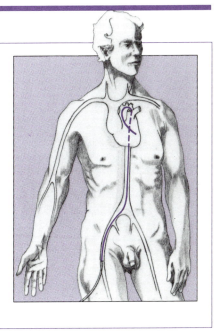

bleeding, keep the patient in bed for 8 to 12 hours, as ordered.

Check the patient's skin color and temperature. Look for a peripheral pulse distal to the puncture site.

If the catheter was inserted into the brachial artery or antecubital vein, keep the arm straight for at least 3 hours. Discourage the patient from using the affected arm for at least 12 hours.

If the femoral artery or vein was used, keep the patient flat for the first 3 hours after the procedure. Keep the affected leg straight for at least 6 hours, immobilizing it by placing a sandbag over the insertion site. Make sure the patient understands that being active, straining, sitting up without assistance, or lifting his head from the bed involves using his abdominal muscles, which puts pressure on the groin and may cause bleeding. If he has to cough

or use the bedpan, tell him to apply pressure to the puncture site.

Regardless of the catheter insertion site, monitor the patient's urine output carefully — especially if he has impaired renal function. Monitor his serum creatinine level for 2 days, looking for signs of renal insufficiency caused by the dye. Consult with the doctor about resuming medications withheld before the test and administer analgesics, as ordered.

Unless the patient is scheduled for surgery, encourage him to drink fluids, especially those high in potassium, such as orange juice. Doing so will help him excrete the contrast medium, and the potassium will help counteract the contrast medium's diuretic effects.

Schedule a posttest ECG to check for possible myocardial damage.

(*Text continues on page 182.*)

Managing cardiac catheterization problems

COMPLICATION AND POSSIBLE CAUSES	SIGNS AND SYMPTOMS	NURSING INTERVENTIONS
Left- or right-side catheterization		
Myocardial infarction • Emotional stress induced by procedure • Blood clot dislodged by catheter tip traveling to a coronary artery (left-side catheterization only) • Air embolism	• Chest pain, possibly radiating to left arm, back, or jaw • Arrhythmias • Diaphoresis, restlessness, anxiety • Thready pulse • Fever • Peripheral cyanosis, causing cool skin	• Give oxygen or medications, as ordered. • Monitor patient continuously, as ordered. • Keep resuscitation equipment available.
Arrhythmias • Cardiac tissue irritated by catheter	• Irregular heartbeat • Irregular apical pulse • Palpitations	• Monitor patient continuously, as ordered. • Administer antiarrhythmic, if ordered.
Cardiac tamponade • Perforation of heart wall by catheter	• Sudden shock • Arrhythmias • Increased heart rate • Decreased blood pressure • Chest pain • Diaphoresis and cyanosis • Distant heart sounds	• Give oxygen, if ordered. • Prepare patient for emergency surgery, if ordered. • Monitor patient continuously, as ordered. • Keep emergency equipment available.
Infection (systemic) • Poor aseptic technique • Catheter contaminated during manufacturing, storage, or use	• Fever • Increased pulse rate • Chills and tremor • Unstable blood pressure	• Collect urine, sputum, and blood samples for culture, as ordered. • Monitor vital signs.
Pulmonary edema • Excessive fluid administration	• Early stage: tachycardia, tachypnea, dependent crackles, diastolic (S_3) gallop • Acute stage: dyspnea; rapid, noisy respirations; cough with frothy, blood-tinged sputum; cyanosis with cold, clammy skin; tachycardia; hypertension	• Administer oxygen, as ordered. • Give medications (digitalis, diuretic, morphine), as ordered. • Restrict fluids and insert an indwelling urinary catheter. • Monitor patient continuously, as ordered. • Maintain patient's airway and keep him in semi-Fowler's position. • Apply rotating tourniquets, as ordered. • Keep resuscitation equipment available.

Managing cardiac catheterization problems *(continued)*

COMPLICATION AND POSSIBLE CAUSES	SIGNS AND SYMPTOMS	NURSING INTERVENTIONS
Left- or right-side catheterization		
Hypovolemia • Diuresis from angiography contrast medium	• Increased urine output • Hypotension	• Replace fluids by giving patient one or two glasses of water every hour, or maintain I.V. infusion rate of 150 to 200 ml/hour, as ordered. • Monitor fluid intake and output closely. • Monitor vital signs.
Hematoma or bleeding at insertion site • Vein or artery damage at insertion site	• Bloody dressing • Limb swelling • Decreased blood pressure • Increased heart rate	• Elevate limb and apply direct manual pressure. • When bleeding stops, apply a pressure bandage. • If bleeding continues or if vital signs are unstable, notify doctor.
Reaction to contrast medium • Allergy to iodine	• Fever • Agitation • Hives • Itching • Decreased urine output, indicating kidney failure • Nausea • Rashes	• Administer antihistamine to relieve itching, as ordered. • Administer diuretic to treat kidney failure, as ordered. • Administer anti-inflammatory agent, as ordered. • Monitor fluid intake and output closely.
Infection at insertion site • Poor aseptic technique	• Swelling, warmth, redness, and soreness at site • Purulent discharge at site	• Obtain drainage specimen for culture. • Clean site, and apply antimicrobial ointment, if ordered. Apply sterile gauze pad. • Review and improve aseptic technique.
Left-side catheterization		
Arterial embolus or thrombus in limb • Injury to artery during catheter insertion, causing blood clot • Plaque dislodged from artery wall by catheter	• Slow or faint pulse distal to insertion site • Loss of warmth, sensation, and color in arm or leg distal to insertion site	• Notify doctor, who may perform an arteriotomy and Fogarty catheterization to remove embolus or thrombus. • Protect affected arm or leg from pressure. Keep it at room temperature, and maintain it at a level or slightly dependent position. • Administer a vasodilator, such as papaverine, to relieve painful vasospasm, if ordered. *(continued)*

Managing cardiac catheterization problems *(continued)*

COMPLICATION AND POSSIBLE CAUSES	SIGNS AND SYMPTOMS	NURSING INTERVENTIONS
Left-side catheterization *(continued)*		
Cerebrovascular accident • Blood clot or plaque dislodged by catheter tip travels to brain	• Hemiplegia • Aphasia • Lethargy • Decreased level of consciousness	• Monitor vital signs closely. • Administer oxygen, as ordered. • Keep suctioning equipment nearby.
Right-side catheterization		
Thrombophlebitis • Vein damaged during catheter insertion	• Hard, sore, cordlike, warm vein • Red line above catheter insertion site • Swelling at insertion site	• Elevate arm or leg, and apply warm, wet compresses. • Administer anticoagulant or fibrinolytic drug, as ordered.
Pulmonary embolism • Blood clot or plaque dislodged by catheter tip travels to lungs	• Shortness of breath • Tachypnea • Increased heart rate • Chest pain	• Place patient in high Fowler's position. • Administer oxygen, if ordered. • Monitor vital signs.
Vagal response • Vagus nerve endings irritated in sinoatrial node, atrial muscle tissue, or atrioventricular junction • Complete heart block	• Hypotension • Decreased heart rate • Nausea	• Monitor heart rate closely. • Administer atropine, if ordered. • Keep patient supine and quiet. • Give liquids.

Normal results

Cardiac catheterization should reveal normal heart chamber size and configuration, wall motion and thickness, direction of blood flow, and valve function. The coronary arteries should appear smooth and regular with no narrowing. A normal ejection fraction (more than 55%) indicates a decreased risk during cardiac surgery.

Abnormal results

Nearly all types of congenital or acquired intracardiac conditions or defects—including CAD, valvular

heart disease, septal defects (atrial and ventricular), ventricular aneurysm, left ventricular enlargement, cardiac tumors, and pericardial constriction—can be detected, evaluated, and documented by cardiac catheterization.

Nursing implications of abnormal results

If the test shows heart disease or a defect, support the patient emotionally. Reinforce the doctor's explanations of the problem and the care required. Answer the patient's questions. If the test indicates a need for cardiac surgery, prepare the patient physically and emotionally.

Cerebrospinal fluid analysis

A clear substance circulating in the subarachnoid space, cerebrospinal fluid (CSF) has several vital functions. It protects the brain and spinal cord from injury and transports products of neurosecretion, cellular biosynthesis, and cellular metabolism through the central nervous system (CNS).

Most commonly, a doctor obtains three CSF samples by lumbar puncture between the third and fourth lumbar vertebrae. If a patient has an infection at this site, lumbar puncture is contraindicated, and the doctor may instead perform a cisternal puncture. If a patient has increased intracranial pressure, the doctor must remove the CSF with extreme caution because the removal of fluid causes a rapid reduction in pressure, which could trigger brain stem herniation. The doctor may instead perform a ventricular puncture on this patient. CSF samples may also be obtained during other neurologic tests—myelography or pneumoencephalography, for instance.

During the procedure, the doctor records CSF pressure and checks the appearance of the samples. Laboratory personnel then perform a quantitative analysis of CSF for protein, glucose, and white and red blood cells, as well as serologic tests, such as the Venereal Disease Research Laboratory test for neurosyphilis. Also in the laboratory, culture and sensitivity tests are performed. Electrolyte analysis and a Gram stain may be done as supplementary tests. The chloride level is particularly useful if a patient has an abnormal serum electrolyte level or a CSF infection, or if he's receiving hyperosmolar agents.

Purpose
• To measure CSF pressure to help detect an obstruction of CSF circulation
• To aid in diagnosing viral or bacterial meningitis, and subarachnoid or intracranial hemorrhage, tumors, and abscesses
• To aid in diagnosing neurosyphilis and chronic CNS infections.

Procedure-related nursing care
Besides performing the nursing care discussed in the chapter introduction, take the following specific measures.

Before the procedure. Tell the patient to remain still and breathe normally during the procedure because movement and hyperventilation can alter pressure readings and cause injury. Following these instructions will also reduce his risk of headache—the most common adverse effect of a lumbar puncture.

Just before the procedure, obtain a lumbar puncture tray. Place the labeled tubes at the bedside, making sure the labels are numbered sequentially, and include the patient's name, date, and room number as well as any laboratory instructions.

During the procedure. If you're assisting with the procedure, position the patient as directed—usually, on his side at the edge of the bed with his knees drawn up as far as possible. This position allows full flexion of the spine and easy access to the lumbar subarachnoid space. Place a

Cerebrospinal fluid analysis: Interpreting abnormal results

ELEMENT	ABNORMAL RESULT	POSSIBLE CAUSES
Cerebrospinal fluid (CSF) pressure	• Increase • Decrease	• Increased intracranial pressure from hemorrhage, tumor, or edema caused by trauma • Spinal subarachnoid obstruction above puncture site
Appearance	• Cloudy • Xantho-chromic • Bloody • Brown • Orange	• Infection • Elevated protein level or red blood cell (RBC) breakdown • Subarachnoid, intracerebral, or intraventricular hemorrhage; spinal cord obstruction; traumatic tap • Meningeal melanoma • Systemic carotenemia
Protein	• Marked increase • Marked decrease	• Tumor, trauma, hemorrhage, diabetes mellitus, polyneuritis, blood in CSF • Rapid CSF production
Gamma globulin	• Increase	• Demyelinating disease (such as multiple sclerosis), neurosyphilis, Guillain-Barré syndrome
Glucose	• Increase • Decrease	• Systemic hyperglycemia • Systemic hypoglycemia, bacterial or fungal infection, meningitis, mumps, postsubarachnoid hemorrhage
Cell count	• Increase in white blood cell count • RBCs present	• Meningitis, acute infection, onset of chronic illness, tumor, abscess, infarction, demyelinating disease (such as multiple sclerosis) • Hemorrhage or traumatic tap
Serologic tests	• Reactive	• Neurosyphilis
Chloride	• Decrease	• Infected meninges (tuberculosis or meningitis)
Gram stain	• Gram-positive or gram-negative organisms	• Bacterial meningitis

small pillow under the patient's head and bend his head forward so his chin touches his chest. Help him hold this position during the procedure. Stand in front of him and place one hand around his neck and the other around his knees.

If the doctor wants the patient sitting, have him sit on the edge of the bed and lower his chest and head toward his knees. Help the patient maintain this position throughout the procedure.

Monitor the patient for signs of adverse reactions, such as elevated pulse rate, pallor, or clammy skin.

Make sure the samples are placed in the appropriately labeled tubes. Record the collection time on the test request form, then send the form and the labeled samples to the laboratory immediately.

After the procedure. After a lumbar puncture, the patient usually lies flat for 8 hours. Some doctors, however, allow a 30-degree elevation of the head of the bed. Encourage the patient to drink plenty of fluids, and remind him that raising his head may cause a headache. If he develops a headache, administer an analgesic, as ordered.

Check the puncture site for redness, swelling, drainage, CSF leakage, and hematoma every hour for the first 4 hours, then every 4 hours for the next 20 hours. Monitor the patient's level of consciousness (LOC), pupillary reaction, and vital signs. Also observe him for signs and symptoms of complications of the lumbar puncture, such as meningitis, cerebellar tonsillar herniation, and medullary compression.

Normal results
Normal CSF pressure ranges from 50 to 180 mm H_2O. The CSF should appear clear and colorless.

Normal protein content ranges between 15 and 45 mg/dl; normal gamma globulin levels, between 3% and 12% of total protein. Glucose levels should range between 45 and 85 mg/dl, which is two-thirds of the blood glucose level. The CSF should contain 0 to 5 white blood cells per microliter and no red blood cells. All serologic tests should be nonreactive.

The chloride level should be 118 to 130 mEq/liter. And the Gram stain should reveal no organisms.

Abnormal results
For a listing of abnormal results and their possible causes, see *Cerebrospinal fluid analysis: Interpreting abnormal results.*

Nursing implications of abnormal results
If the test shows elevated CSF pressure, assess the patient's neurologic status every 15 minutes for 4 hours. If you detect a decreasing LOC or pupillary reaction, notify the doctor immediately. Expect to administer an osmotic diuretic, as ordered. If the patient is stable after the first 4 hours, assess him every hour for 2 hours, then once every 4 hours or according to the pretest schedule.

Electrocardiography

The most common procedure for evaluating cardiac status, electrocardiography graphically records the conduction, magnitude, and duration of the heart's electrical potential. To perform this test, you'll place 10 electrodes on the patient's limbs and chest. These electrodes then create 12 distinct views (or leads) of the heart's electrical activity.

The six limb leads, which reflect electrical potential in the heart's vertical plane, include leads I, II, III, aV_R (augmented vector right), aV_L (augmented vector left), and aV_F (augmented vector foot). The six chest (or precordial) leads, which provide information on the heart's horizontal plane, are called leads V_1, V_2, V_3, V_4, V_5, and V_6.

Limb leads I, II, and III are bipolar, meaning they require two electrodes to measure electrical activity. Limb leads aV_R, aV_L, and aV_F and the six precordial leads are unipolar. This means they need only a positive electrode; the negative pole of the lead, which is in the center of the heart, is calculated by the electrocardiograph (ECG).

For the limb leads, you'll place

electrodes on the arms and legs, with the ground lead on the right leg. Limb lead I measures the electrical potential between the left and right arms; limb lead II, between the left leg and right arm; and limb lead III, between the left leg and left arm. Leads aV_R, aV_L, and aV_F measure electrical potential between one augmented limb lead and the electrical midpoint of the other two leads (determined electronically by the ECG). For information on placing the chest electrodes, refer to *Electrode positions for precordial leads.*

For all 12 leads, the electrical potentials are transmitted to the ECG, which amplifies and graphically displays them on a strip chart recorder. The graphic display, or tracing, usually consists of the P wave, the QRS complex, and the T wave. The P wave shows atrial depolarization; the QRS complex shows ventricular depolarization; and the T wave shows ventricular repolarization.

Purpose
• To help identify primary conduction abnormalities, cardiac arrhythmias, cardiac hypertrophy, pericarditis, electrolyte imbalances, myocardial ischemia, and the site and extent of a myocardial infarction (MI)
• To monitor recovery from an MI
• To evaluate the effectiveness of cardiac medication — such as glycosides, antiarrhythmics, antihypertensives, and vasodilators
• To observe pacemaker performance.

Procedure-related nursing care
Besides performing the nursing care discussed in the chapter introduction, take the following specific measures.

Before the procedure. Tell the patient to relax, lie still, and breathe normally during the test. Advise him not to talk during the test because the sound of his voice may distort the ECG tracing. Check his history for cardiac drugs, and note any current therapy on the test request form.

During the procedure. Place the patient in the supine position. (If he's orthopneic, place him in semi-Fowler's position.) Tell him not to touch the bed's metal handrail or allow his feet to touch the footboard because this can cause current leakage that distorts the ECG tracing.

How you perform the procedure will depend on whether you're using a single-channel or a multi-channel ECG.

With a *single-channel ECG*, you can record only one lead at a time. To use this machine, turn it on and set the lead selector to the standby mode to warm up the stylus machine. Check the paper supply and center the stylus on the paper.

Prepare the electrode sites. If necessary, clip or shave the hair around the sites. Then clean them with alcohol and allow them to dry completely. Open the electrode disk packets and check that the disks have adequate gel. If the gel has dried on any of the disks, replace them.

Position the limb electrodes on flat, fleshy, hairless sites on the arms and legs — usually the inner forearm and the inner calf just above the ankle. Position the chest electrodes on the precordial lead sites. Then attach the electrode cables, or lead wires, to the four limb disks.

Turn the lead selector to lead I. Write the lead number on the paper strip, or push the marking button on

Electrode positions for precordial leads

Place the electrodes as follows:

- V_1: fourth intercostal space (ICS), right sternal border
- V_2: fourth ICS, left sternal border
- V_3: midway between V_2 and V_4

- V_4: fifth ICS, left midclavicular line
- V_5: fifth ICS, left anterior axillary line
- V_6: fifth ICS, left midaxillary line

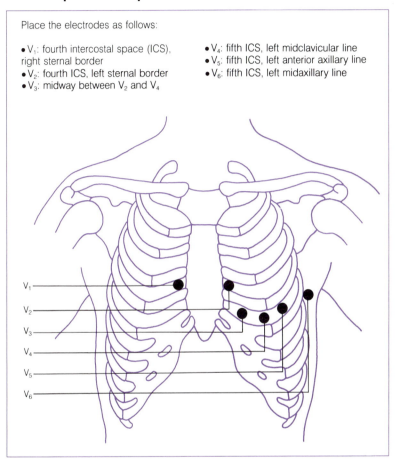

the machine to identify the lead with a code indicating the waveform for that lead. Record for 3 to 5 seconds and then return the machine to the standby mode. Repeat this procedure for leads II, III, aV_R, aV_L, and aV_F. Then turn the lead selector to a neutral position before running precordial leads V_1 through V_6. This prevents the stylus from swinging wildly and possibly damaging the paper.

Next, connect a lead wire to the electrode at the V_1 position. Turn the lead selector to the V_1 position and record for 3 to 5 seconds. Then return the lead selector to the neutral position, remove the lead wire from the V_1 electrode, and attach it to the V_2 electrode. Turn the selector to V_2 and record. Repeat this procedure through lead V_6, always turning the selector to the neutral position before moving the lead wire.

After completing V_6, run a rhythm strip on lead II for at least 6 seconds. Now assess the quality of the whole series and repeat individual lead tracings as needed.

If you're using a *multi-channel 12-lead ECG*, you'll record all 12 leads at one time. First, prepare the ECG and the electrode sites and position the electrodes as you would for a single-channel ECG. Then attach the lead wires to all the electrodes, including the six precordial lead electrodes, before making a recording. You don't need to reset the lead selector or reposition the leads during the test.

After the procedure. After using the single- or multi-channel ECG, disconnect the equipment and remove the electrodes. Then wash any conductive gel from the patient's skin with a damp cloth.

Normal results

Each of the 12 leads should show normal positive and negative ECG deflections.

The limb lead II waveform, known as the rhythm strip, depicts the heart's rhythm more clearly than any other waveform and is parallel to the wave of depolarization. In this lead, the P wave normally doesn't exceed 2.5 mm (0.25 mV) in height or last longer than 0.11 second. The PR interval (which includes the P wave plus the PR segment) persists for 0.12 to 0.20 second for cardiac rates over 60 beats/minute. The QT interval varies with the cardiac rate. And the QRS interval should last 0.06 to 0.10 second.

In leads V_1 through V_6, R wave voltage shouldn't exceed 27 mm.

Abnormal results

An abnormal ECG may show an MI,

right or left ventricular hypertrophy, right or left atrial hypertrophy, arrhythmias, right or left bundle-branch block, ischemia, conduction defects, pericarditis, electrolyte abnormalities such as hyperkalemia, and the effects of cardioactive drugs.

Nursing implications of abnormal results

If the ECG results indicate an arrhythmia, explain the importance of prompt treatment and intervene, as ordered.

If the test was done to monitor the evolution of an MI, or another problem was identified, offer the patient support and reinforce the doctor's explanation. Stress the importance of following the prescribed care plan.

Electroencephalography

For this test, an examiner attaches electrodes to the patient's scalp to record the portion of the brain's electrical activity that reaches the scalp's surface. The electroencephalograph (EEG) receives the impulses, magnifies them 1 million times, and then records them as brain waves on moving strips of paper. The recording is used to evaluate the basic waveforms, the symmetry of cerebral activity, transient discharges, and responses to stimulation. Some waveforms will appear irregular, while others will show recurring patterns.

In a patient who has a seizure disorder, an EEG may help identify the specific type of seizure, such as generalized tonic-clonic or complex partial. The test can also be used to help diagnose other disorders, such as intracranial lesions.

Usually, this test is performed in a room designed to eliminate electrical interference and minimize distractions. A portable unit, however, may be used to perform an EEG at bedside, particularly to test an unstable patient or to aid in diagnosing brain death.

Purpose
• To determine the presence and type of seizures
• To aid in diagnosing intracranial lesions, such as abscesses and tumors
• To evaluate the brain's electrical activity in metabolic disease, head injury, meningitis, encephalitis, mental retardation, and psychological disorders
• To aid in diagnosing brain death.

Procedure-related nursing care
Besides performing the nursing care discussed in the chapter introduction, take the following specific measures.

Before the procedure. Tell the patient that he'll be positioned comfortably on a bed or a reclining chair. Explain that electrodes will be attached to his scalp but that they won't shock him. Usually, flat electrodes will be applied with a special paste. However, if needle electrodes will be used, explain that he'll feel a pricking sensation on insertion.

Advise him that before the procedure begins, he'll have to close his eyes, relax, and remain still. Do your best to allay his fears because mental tension can affect the brain-wave patterns.

Tell the patient not to drink fluids that contain caffeine, such as coffee and cola, before the test. But be sure he doesn't skip a meal; doing so can cause relative hypoglycemia

and alter brain-wave patterns. Also, tell him to wash and dry his hair thoroughly, leaving no traces of hair sprays, creams, or oils.

As ordered, withhold anticonvulsants, tranquilizers, barbiturates, and other sedatives for 24 to 48 hours before the test. If ordered, administer a sedative to an infant or a young child to prevent crying and restlessness during the test.

If a sleep EEG has been ordered, keep the patient awake most of the night before the test, letting him sleep only between midnight and 4 a.m. If he can't sleep for the test, he may receive a sedative.

During the procedure. If you're present for the procedure, observe the patient for seizure activity. Note any seizure patterns, and be prepared to provide assistance in case of a severe seizure. Have suction equipment and diazepam for I.V. injection nearby.

After the procedure. Help the patient remove the electrode paste from his hair, using acetone. Consult with his doctor about resuming any medication therapy that was discontinued before the test. If the patient received a sedative before the test, take safety precautions, such as raising the side rails and keeping the bed lowered.

Normal results
The brain waves should have normal characteristics, amplitude, and frequency.

Abnormal results
EEGs can help diagnose seizure disorders; intracranial lesions, such as tumors and abscesses; vascular lesions, such as cerebral infarcts; metabolic disorders; inflammatory processes, such as meningitis or en-

cephalitis; and brain death.

Nursing implications of abnormal results

If the test results indicate a seizure disorder, support the patient emotionally and take the appropriate seizure precautions. Teach the patient about his disorder. Also, as appropriate, explain that he'll need to take a medication to control seizure activity.

If the test confirms the presence of a lesion, prepare the patient for further testing and possible surgery. Tell him about other diagnostic studies that can be performed, such as magnetic resonance imaging or a computed tomography scan.

If the test reveals diffuse brain abnormalities, explain how the findings relate to the patient's behavior. If necessary, discuss cerebral physiology and function to help the patient understand the implications of the findings.

Magnetic resonance imaging

Even though the full range of its clinical applications hasn't yet been established, magnetic resonance imaging (MRI) has already proven to be a valuable tool for neurologic and cardiovascular diagnosis. A safe, noninvasive imaging technique, MRI allows the examiner to see through bone and view fluid-filled soft tissue in great detail. It provides sharp differentiation between healthy and diseased tissues as well as a clear view of arteries and veins. MRI provides greater tissue discrimination than computed tomography scanning — without the risks associated

with ionizing radiation and injected contrast media. (Contrast media, however, are now being used for MRI brain studies.)

MRI relies on the magnetic properties of the atom to develop its images. Hydrogen, the most abundant and magnetically sensitive of the body's atoms, is most commonly used for MRI studies. The MRI scanner uses a powerful magnetic field and radio-frequency energy to produce images based on the hydrogen (or water) content of body tissues. These high-resolution, three-dimensional images can be recorded on film or magnetic tape for permanent storage.

MRI shouldn't be used on patients with intracranial aneurysm clips, orthopedic screws, or ferrous metal implants (such as pacemakers or insulin pumps). Nor should patients requiring life-support equipment undergo MRI because the equipment won't function properly within a magnetic field.

Purpose
● To aid in diagnosing intracranial and spinal lesions as well as cardiovascular and soft-tissue abnormalities.

Procedure-related nursing care
Besides performing the nursing care discussed in the chapter introduction, take the following specific measures.

Explain to the patient that he'll go to the scanner room, where he'll be placed on a narrow, padded, nonmetallic stretcher that's designed to fit into the scanner tunnel. Then he'll be wheeled into the tunnel.

Tell the patient that he'll have to remain still for 5- to 20-minute intervals while in the tunnel. If he has claustrophobic tendencies, ask the doctor to order a sedative.

Assure the patient that the test doesn't expose him to radiation and that he'll feel no pain. Explain that during the test he may hear the machine make metallic thumping noises that sound like drumbeats. If he thinks this will bother him, he can ask for earplugs.

Check the patient's history to find out if he has any metal in his body. Even a small piece can cause serious injury. For example, a metal fleck in the eye can cause retinal hemorrhage during MRI.

Because the test can take up to 1½ hours, advise the patient to void before it begins. A hospitalized patient should wear a loose-fitting hospital gown. Tell an outpatient to wear comfortable clothing. Explain to the patient that he must remove all jewelry because it may be damaged by the strong magnetic field. Tell him someone will check to make sure he has removed all metal objects just before he enters the scanner room.

Normal results

The image should show normal anatomic and biochemical tissue details in any plane, without bone interference.

Abnormal results

MRI can detect tumors, abscesses, and fractures; demyelinating diseases, such as multiple sclerosis; intracranial problems, such as cerebral edema, plaque formations, infarctions, tumors, blood clots, hemorrhage, and aneurysms; and cardiovascular problems, such as cardiac valve abnormalities, aortic atherosclerosis, and ventricular hypertrophy.

Nursing implications of abnormal results

If the test results reveal a problem, you'll need to support the patient emotionally and reinforce the doctor's explanation of the problem and required care.

Papanicolaou test

A cytologic evaluation, the Papanicolaou (Pap) test is widely known for its use in the early detection of cervical cancer. It's also used to detect inflammatory disorders and to assess a patient's response to hormonal treatment, although this entry focuses on its use in detecting cervical cancer. The most common specimen consists of cervical scrapings, although vaginal scrapings can be used to assess the effects of hormonal treatment. The Pap test can show cell maturity, metabolic activity, and morphologic variations of the specimen.

The American Cancer Society recommends a cervical Pap test every 3 years for women between ages 20 and 40 who aren't in a high-risk category for cervical cancer and who've had three previous negative Pap tests. Annual tests (or tests performed at intervals ordered by the patient's doctor) are recommended for women over age 40, for those in a high-risk category, and for those who've had at least one positive test.

Purpose

- To detect malignant cells
- To detect inflammatory tissue changes
- To assess patient response to chemotherapy and radiation therapy
- To detect viral, fungal and, occasionally, parasitic invasion
- To assess the effects of hormonal treatment.

Performing a Pap test

A specially trained nurse can perform a Pap test by following these steps.

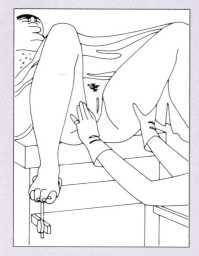

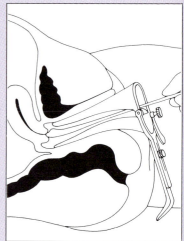

Ask the patient to disrobe from the waist down. Put on gloves. Have the patient lie on the examining table and drape her from the waist down. Ask her to place her heels in the stirrups and then slide her buttocks to the edge of the table. Adjust the drape, as necessary.

To ease the insertion of the unlubricated speculum, first place it under warm running water. Ask the patient to spread her knees apart. Insert the speculum into the vagina and expose the cervix by opening the speculum blades. Then lock the blades in place. Insert a saline-moistened Pap spatula through the speculum and scrape secretions from the cervix and endocervical canal by rotating the spatula 360 degrees.

Procedure-related nursing care
Besides performing the nursing care discussed in the chapter introduction, take the following specific measures. Stress the importance of the test as a way of detecting cancer early, when it commonly produces no symptoms and is still curable.

Explain to the patient that the test won't be done while she's menstruating. The ideal time is midway through her menstrual cycle. Advise her not to douche or insert vaginal medications for 24 hours before the test. Doing so can wash away cellular deposits and change the vaginal pH.

Note any pertinent patient history information on the laboratory slip. If the patient appears anxious, be supportive and tell her that test results will be available within a few days.

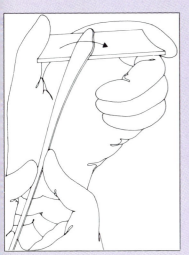

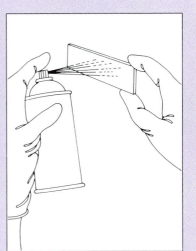

After you obtain the secretions, remove the spatula and prepare a specimen slide. Spread the secretions across the top of a microscopic slide, according to laboratory recommendation.

Immediately apply a fixative to the slide. In most cases, you'll spray on a commercial fixative, as shown. Or you can immerse the slide in a solution of 95% ethyl alcohol. With either method, label the specimen appropriately, including the date, the patient's age, the date of her last menstrual period, and the collection site and method used. Unlock and withdraw the speculum and help the patient to a sitting position.

Just before the test, have her empty her bladder.

Usually, a doctor performs the Pap test with a nurse assisting him. However, a specially trained nurse can also perform the procedure (see *Performing a Pap test*).

If cervical bleeding occurs after the test, give the patient a sanitary napkin. Tell her when to return for her next Pap test.

Normal results
No malignant cells or other abnormalities should be present.

Abnormal results
Usually, malignant cells have relatively large nuclei and only small amounts of cytoplasm. They show abnormal nuclear chromatin patterns and marked variation in size, shape, and staining properties. They

may have prominent nucleoli.

A Pap smear may be graded in different ways, so review your laboratory's reporting format. The following system is the traditional specimen classification method:
• *Class I*—normal pattern; absence of atypical or abnormal cells
• *Class II*—benign abnormality; atypical, but nonmalignant, cells present
• *Class III*—atypical cells consistent with dysplasia
• *Class IV*—suggestive of, but inconclusive for, cancer
• *Class V*—conclusive for cancer.

Many clinicians prefer to classify Pap test results according to the following descriptive terminology:
• normal
• metaplasia
• inflammation
• minimal atypia—koilocytosis
• mild dysplasia (CIN I)
• moderate dysplasia (CIN II)
• severe dysplasia—carcinoma in situ (CIN III)
• invasive carcinoma.

Nursing implications of abnormal results
If a Pap test is positive or suggests cancer, support the patient emotionally. Anticipate a cervical biopsy to confirm the diagnosis. Reinforce the doctor's explanation of the test results and further tests.

Pulmonary function tests

A group of dynamic studies, pulmonary function tests (PFTs) evaluate ventilatory function. To obtain results for most of these tests, you'll use either a direct spirometric measurement or certain calculations based on spirometric measurements.

Of the five tests used to determine lung volume, tidal volume (VT) and expiratory reserve volume (ERV) are direct spirometric measurements. Minute volume (MV), inspiratory reserve volume (IRV), and residual volume (RV) are calculated from the results of other PFTs.

The tests used to measure lung capacity—forced vital capacity (FVC), flow-volume curve, forced expiratory volume (FEV), and maximal voluntary ventilation (MVV)—are direct spirometric measurements. Vital capacity (VC), inspiratory capacity (IC), functional residual capacity (FRC), and peak expiratory flow (PEF) can be measured directly or calculated. Total lung capacity (TLC) and forced expiratory flow ($FEF_{25\% \text{ to } 75\%}$) are calculated from other spirometric results. (See *Reading a spirogram*, opposite, and *Interpreting pulmonary function tests*, pages 196 to 198.)

Other PFTs, which aren't discussed here, require specialized equipment and are usually performed on patients with identified pulmonary disease. These tests measure carbon dioxide response, peak flow, and uniformity of ventilation.

Purpose
• To determine the cause of dyspnea
• To assess the effectiveness of therapy
• To distinguish obstructive from restrictive disorders
• To estimate the degree of pulmonary dysfunction
• To establish baseline pulmonary function for future comparison
• To provide objective evidence of subjective symptoms
• To document a disability
• To detect early signs of respiratory impairment in asymptomatic patients.

Reading a spirogram

The plotting of a spirogram, or lung signature, is based on the patient's tidal volume (VT) and his maximum inspiration (A) and expiration (B) capabilities. Together, these constitute vital capacity (VC). After they've been plotted, a spirogram can be used to calculate inspiratory reserve volume (IRV), expiratory reserve volume (ERV), residual volume (RV), inspiratory capacity (IC), functional residual capacity (FRC), and total lung capacity (TLC), as shown below. (In the illustration, the gray area indicates normal breathing.)

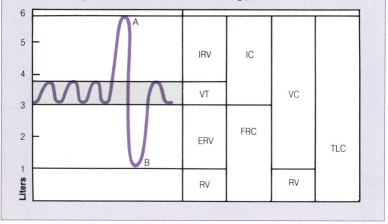

Procedure-related nursing care

Besides performing the nursing care discussed in the chapter introduction, take the following specific measures.

Before the procedure. Tell the patient where the test will be performed and who'll administer it. It may take place in a pulmonary laboratory, a doctor's office, or at the bedside using a portable spirometer. Explain that he'll have to wear a nose clip during the procedure. Tell him that although the test is painless, it may prove tiring. Assure him that he'll be allowed to rest as necessary. Emphasize that the test's accuracy depends on his cooperation.

Instruct the patient not to eat a heavy meal before the test. If his treatment regimen is being as-

sessed, administer his medications, as ordered. Otherwise, expect to withhold bronchodilators. Steroids are rarely withheld because their effects wear off so slowly.

Just before the test, have the patient void. Tell him to loosen any restrictive clothing. If he wears dentures, tell him to leave them in place because they'll help keep his mouth sealed around the mouthpiece of the spirometer.

During the procedure. A respiratory therapist usually administers PFTs. If, however, you're administering them, follow these steps.

Seat the patient next to the spirometer and position the nose clip so that he breathes only through his mouth. Air leaks from the nose can

(Text continues on page 198.)

Interpreting pulmonary function tests

MEASUREMENT OF PULMONARY FUNCTION	METHOD OF CALCULATION	IMPLICATIONS
Tidal volume (VT) Amount of air inhaled or exhaled during normal breathing	Determine the spirometric measurement for 10 breaths, then divide by 10.	Decreased VT may indicate restrictive disease and requires further testing, such as complete pulmonary function studies or chest radiography.
Minute volume (MV) Total amount of air breathed per minute	Multiply VT by the respiratory rate.	Normal MV can occur in emphysema. Decreased MV may indicate other diseases, such as pulmonary edema. Increased MV can occur with acidosis, increased carbon dioxide levels, decreased partial pressure of oxygen in arterial blood, and exercise.
Maximum inspiratory pressure (MIP) The amount of pressure generated when attempting to initiate an inhalation	Measure using inspiratory pressure manometer.	Decreased MIP appears in neuromuscular disorders and indicates the need to initiate mechanical ventilation. Improvement can help determine successful weaning.
Inspiratory reserve volume (IRV) Amount of air inspired in excess of normal inspiration	Subtract VT from inspiratory capacity.	Abnormal IRV alone doesn't indicate respiratory dysfunction. IRV decreases during normal exercise.
Expiratory reserve volume (ERV) Amount of air that can be forcibly exhaled beyond VT.	Use direct spirometric measurement.	ERV varies, even in healthy persons, but usually decreases in obese persons.
Residual volume (RV) Amount of air remaining in the lungs after forced expiration	Subtract ERV from functional residual capacity.	RV greater than 35% of total lung capacity (TLC) after maximal expiratory effort may indicate obstructive disease.
Vital capacity (VC) Total volume of air that can be exhaled after maximum inspiration	Use direct spirometric measurement, or add VT, IRV, and ERV.	Normal or increased VC with decreased flow rates may indicate any condition that causes a reduction in functional pulmonary tissue, such as pulmonary edema. Decreased VC with normal or increased flow rates may indicate decreased respiratory effort resulting from neuromuscular diseases, drug overdose, or head injury; decreased thoracic expansion; or limited movement of the diaphragm.
Inspiratory capacity (IC) Amount of air that can be inhaled after normal expiration	Use direct spirometric measurement, or add IRV and VT.	Decreased IC indicates restrictive disease.

Interpreting pulmonary function tests (continued)

MEASUREMENT OF PULMONARY FUNCTION	METHOD OF CALCULATION	IMPLICATIONS
Forced vital capacity (FVC) The amount of air exhaled forcefully and quickly after maximum inspiration	Use direct spirometric measurement; expressed as a percentage of the total volume of gas exhaled.	Decreased FVC indicates flow resistance in the respiratory system from obstructive disease, such as chronic bronchitis, or from restrictive disease, such as pulmonary fibrosis.
Flow-volume curve [also called flow-volume loop] Greatest rate of flow (Vmax) during FVC maneuvers versus lung volume change	Use direct spirometric measurement at 1-second intervals; calculated from flow rates (expressed in liters/second) and lung volume changes (expressed in liters) during maximal inspiratory and expiratory maneuvers.	Decreased flow rates at all volumes during expiration indicate obstructive disease of the small airways, such as emphysema. A plateau of expiratory flow near TLC, a plateau of inspiratory flow at mid-VC, and a square wave pattern through most of VC indicate obstructive disease of the large airways. Normal or increased peak expiratory flow, decreased flow with decreasing lung volumes, and markedly decreased VC indicate restrictive disease.
Forced expiratory volume (FEV) Volume of air expired in the first, second, or third second of FVC maneuver	Use direct spirometric measurement; expressed as a percentage of FVC.	Decreased FEV_1 and increased FEV_2 and FEV_3 may indicate obstructive disease. Decreased or normal FEV_1 may indicate restrictive disease.
Forced expiratory flow ($FEF_{25\% \text{ to } 75\%}$) Average rate of flow during middle half of FVC	Calculate from the flow rate and the time needed for expiration of middle 50% of FVC.	Low $FEF_{25\% \text{ to } 75\%}$ indicates obstructive disease of the small airways.
Peak expiratory flow (PEF) Vmax during forced expiration	Calculate from flow-volume curve or by direct spirometric measurement, using a pneumotachometer or an electronic tachometer with a transducer to convert flow to electrical output display.	Decreased PEF may indicate a mechanical problem, such as upper airway obstruction or obstructive disease. PEF is usually normal in restrictive disease but decreases in severe cases. Because PEF is effort-dependent, it's also low in a person who has poor expiratory effort or doesn't understand the procedure.
Maximal voluntary ventilation (MVV) [also called maximum breathing capacity] Greatest volume of air breathed per unit of time	Use direct spirometric measurement.	Decreased MVV may indicate obstructive disease. Normal or decreased MVV may indicate restrictive disease, such as myasthenia gravis.

(continued)

Interpreting pulmonary function tests (continued)

MEASUREMENT OF PULMONARY FUNCTION	METHOD OF CALCULATION	IMPLICATIONS
Functional residual capacity (FRC) Amount of air remaining in lungs after normal expiration	Measure using body plethysmography or helium dilution technique (this procedure is usually performed by a respiratory therapist).	Increased FRC indicates overdistended lungs, which may result from obstructive disease.
Total lung capacity (TLC) Total volume of the lungs when maximally inflated	Add VT, IRV, ERV, and RV; or add FRC and IC; or add VC and RV.	Low TLC indicates restrictive disease. High TLC indicates overdistended lungs caused by obstructive disease.

decrease the measurements. Have him insert the mouthpiece, which attaches to a hose connected to the test machine. The patient should breathe normally through the mouthpiece until he's comfortable and you've checked for and fixed any leaks.

Next, tell the patient to breathe in as deeply as he can and hold his breath momentarily. Then have him blow into the machine as forcefully, rapidly, and completely as he can until you tell him to stop. Even if he feels as though he has exhaled all the air he can, he should continue until you tell him to stop.

Have him breathe normally through the machine, then repeat the procedure until two measurements come within 10% of each other. This confirms that the patient gave his maximum effort and that his volumes and flows are accurate.

To determine if the patient has reversible obstructive airway disease or to objectively document the efficacy of a bronchodilator, you can repeat the test after the patient has inhaled the medication. Be sure the medication has enough time to take

effect before repeating the test. Also make sure the patient knows he received a bronchodilator and note the medication administration on his chart, so he doesn't receive another dose too soon.

After the procedure. Tell the patient to resume his normal diet. Be sure his test results are documented, especially if he's scheduled for surgery.

Reference values
All reference values are predicted for each patient based on his age, height, and sex. Results are usually expressed as percentages of predicted values. A nomogram showing reference values can be obtained from manufacturers of mechanical spirometers. Reference values are programmed into electronic spirometers. A value of 85% or more of the predicted value is considered normal.

Abnormal results
Generally, volume decreases in restrictive disease, and flow rates decrease in obstructive disease.

Nursing implications
of abnormal results

If the test results indicate respiratory impairment, teach the patient about his care plan. The plan may include avoiding pulmonary irritants such as smoke, taking medications, receiving chest physiotherapy, using proper coughing and breathing techniques, receiving oxygen therapy, using energy conservation techniques, and learning the signs of respiratory failure.

Suggested readings

April, E.W. *Anatomy*, 2nd ed. New York: John Wiley & Sons, 1990.

Campbell, C.D., and Newsome, J.A. "Detecting Life-threatening Arrhythmias," *Nursing90* 20(12):34-39, December 1990.

Cardiopulmonary Emergencies. Springhouse, Pa.: Springhouse Corp., 1991.

Corbett, J.V. *Laboratory Tests and Diagnostic Procedures with Nursing Diagnoses*, 2nd ed. Norwalk, Conn.: Appleton & Lange, 1987.

Diagnostics, 2nd ed. Nurse's Reference Library. Springhouse, Pa.: Springhouse Corp., 1987.

Diagnostic Tests. Nurse's Ready Reference. Springhouse, Pa.: Springhouse Corp., 1991.

Fischbach, F.T. *A Manual of Laboratory Diagnostic Tests*, 3rd ed. Philadelphia: J.B. Lippincott Co., 1988.

Kee, J.L. *Handbook of Laboratory and Diagnostic Tests with Nursing Implications*. Norwalk, Conn.: Appleton & Lange, 1990.

Plankey, E.D., and Knauf, J. "Prep Talk: What Patients Need to Know About Magnetic Resonance Imaging," *AJN* 90(1):27-28, January 1990.

Respiratory Care Handbook. Springhouse, Pa.: Springhouse Corp., 1989.

Speicher, C.E. *The Right Test: A Physician's Guide to Laboratory Medicine.* Philadelphia: W.B. Saunders Co., 1989.

SELF-TEST

Test your knowledge and skills at your own pace by answering the multiple-choice questions on pages 201 to 204. Answers appear on page 204.

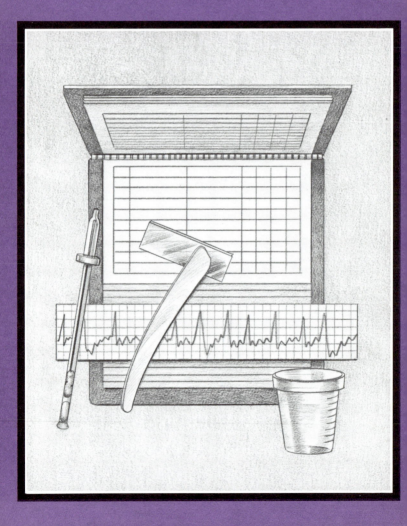

QUESTIONS

1. *You should assess a patient with increased serum aldosterone levels for:*
a. hypotension and hyperkalemia.
b. hypertension and hypokalemia.
c. hypertension and hyponatremia.
d. hypotension and hypernatremia.

2. *You should assess a patient with increased plasma ammonia levels for:*
a. personality changes, confusion, asterixis, lethargy, and stupor (from hepatic coma).
b. gastrointestinal bleeding, seizures, muscle rigidity, and tetany (from liver damage).
c. spider angioma, purpura, hypotension, and bradycardia (from vascular toxicity).
d. oliguria, hypertension, arrhythmias, and muscle weakness (from electrolyte depletion).

3. *Which of the following is true?*
a. Serum and urine amylase levels both rise 7 to 14 days after the onset of acute pancreatitis.
b. Urine amylase levels rise only in response to renal dysfunction, not to acute pancreatitis.
c. Serum amylase levels usually return to normal within 3 days of the onset of acute pancreatitis, but urine amylase levels remain high for 7 to 10 days.
d. Urine amylase levels rise before serum levels in acute pancreatitis.

4. *Your patient's arterial blood gas results include a $PaCO_2 > 45$ mm Hg, a pH < 7.35, and an $HCO_3^- > 26$ mEq/liter. He has:*
a. respiratory alkalosis with renal compensation.
b. respiratory acidosis with renal compensation.
c. metabolic alkalosis with pulmonary compensation.
d. metabolic acidosis with pulmonary compensation.

5. *After you draw a blood sample for a serum bilirubin test, you should:*
a. cover the site with a pressure dressing and ice to prevent bleeding.

b. invert the test tube to delay clotting.
c. take the patient's vital signs to detect hemorrhage.
d. protect the sample from sunlight and ultraviolet light to prevent the bilirubin from breaking down.

6. *What should you do when your patient has an elevated blood urea nitrogen (BUN) level?*
a. Teach him to follow a high-protein diet to replace lost protein.
b. Check the results of his serum enzyme test to find the cause of the elevated BUN level.
c. Assess his level of consciousness (LOC), fluid intake, and urine output.
d. Watch the cardiac monitor for arrhythmias, and monitor his vital signs and respiratory pattern.

7. *Your patient has an elevated serum calcium level. You should:*
a. promote active and passive range-of-motion exercises if he's bedridden.
b. tell him to stop taking digitalis.
c. observe him for Chvostek's sign and tetany.
d. tell him to avoid antacids and laxatives.

8. *Signs and symptoms of a low serum chloride level include:*
a. hypertension, arrhythmias, edema, and fatigue.
b. tetany, muscle hypertonicity, depressed respirations, and hypotension.
c. weakness, tachypnea, stupor, and tachycardia.
d. venous distention, dyspnea, cough, and crackles.

9. *What's the ideal blood cholesterol level for most adults?*
a. between 200 and 240 mg/dl
b. between 240 and 280 mg/dl
c. below 300 mg/dl
d. below 200 mg/dl

10. *After an acute myocardial infarction (MI) or cardiac surgery, you should expect a patient's CPK-MB levels to:*
a. rise in 2 to 4 hours, peak in 12 to 14

hours, and return to normal in 24 to 48 hours.
b. rise in 12 to 14 hours, peak in 48 hours, and return to normal in 72 hours.
c. rise at once, peak in 2 to 4 hours, and return to normal in 24 hours.
d. rise in 1 to 4 hours, peak in 48 hours, and return to normal in 72 hours.

11. *Which test is the best indicator of renal function?*
a. serum aldosterone
b. plasma ammonia
c. serum creatine phosphokinase
d. creatinine clearance

12. *Which result signals diabetes mellitus in a nonpregnant adult?*
a. a fasting plasma glucose level at or above 100 mg/dl on at least three occasions
b. a plasma glucose level at or above 150 mg/dl on at least two occasions
c. a fasting plasma glucose level at or above 140 mg/dl on at least two occasions
d. a fasting plasma glucose level below 110 mg/dl and at least two oral glucose tolerance tests showing a lowered plasma glucose level

13. *When your patient has elevated hemoglobin and hematocrit levels, you should assess him for:*
a. dehydration.
b. anemia.
c. shock.
d. overhydration.

14. *A patient with a positive HIV antibody serum enzyme immunoassay:*
a. has acquired immunodeficiency syndrome (AIDS).
b. will develop AIDS within a year.
c. will need another test, such as the Western blot, to rule out a false-positive result.
d. will need another test, such as the aspartate aminotransferase test, to monitor the progress of the disease.

15. *A flipped LDH means your patient:*
a. needs lifelong care for muscular dystrophy.
b. may have angina, although tissue necrosis hasn't occurred.

c. needs immediate heart surgery.
d. has probably suffered an MI.

16. *Which statement about the lipoprotein-cholesterol fractionation test is correct?*
a. An increased high-density lipoprotein (HDL) level indicates significant atherosclerosis.
b. An increased low-density lipoprotein (LDL) level increases the risk of coronary artery disease.
c. A decreased HDL level signals chronic hepatitis.
d. A decreased LDL level indicates significant heart damage.

17. *Assess a patient with a platelet count below 50,000/mm³ for:*
a. spontaneous bleeding.
b. altered LOC.
c. iron deficiency.
d. severe infection.

18. *Which test definitively diagnoses potassium imbalance in a patient with an abnormal serum potassium level?*
a. serum sodium
b. urine potassium
c. urine sodium
d. electrocardiogram

19. *If your patient undergoes a serum protein electrophoresis test that shows abnormal gamma globulin levels, you should:*
a. assess him for bleeding.
b. protect him from infection.
c. monitor his cardiac status.
d. provide him with a low-protein, high-fat diet.

20. *Notify the doctor if a patient receiving an oral anticoagulant has:*
a. a prothrombin time (PT) three times the control level.
b. a PT one and a half times the control level.
c. an activated partial thromboplastin time (APTT) of 30 seconds.
d. an APTT of 36 seconds.

21. *Insufficient water intake can result in which of the following test results?*
a. a decreased serum sodium level
b. an increased serum sodium level

c. a decreased hematocrit level
d. a decreased white blood cell (WBC) count

22. *Which of the following should a patient with an increased serum uric acid level avoid because of its high purine content?*
a. bread
b. apples
c. scallops
d. milk

23. *If your patient has an increased WBC count, you should:*
a. protect him from infection.
b. assess him for infection and inflammation.
c. protect him from hazards that could result in hemorrhage.
d. assess him for bleeding.

24. *Which of the following is* not *found in normal urine?*
a. hemoglobin
b. creatinine
c. aldosterone
d. potassium

25. *After angiography, you should always:*
a. enforce bed rest for 48 hours.
b. restrict fluids for 24 hours.
c. assess the injection site for bleeding and hematomas.
d. administer an antihistamine to prevent an allergic reaction.

26. *How does digital subtraction angiography (DSA) differ from conventional angiography?*
a. DSA always requires an I.V. injection of a contrast medium.
b. DSA doesn't use a computer to enhance its images.
c. DSA images of the vasculature aren't as clear.
d. DSA never requires an I.V. injection of a contrast medium.

27. *The quickest, most accurate test for cholecystitis is:*
a. oral cholecystography.
b. T-tube cholangiography.
c. a gallbladder computed tomography scan.
d. a liver-spleen scan.

28. *Throat cultures are commonly used to isolate and identify:*
a. alpha-hemolytic streptococci.
b. *Neisseria* species.
c. diphtheroids.
d. group A beta-hemolytic streptococci.

29. *After your patient has a percutaneous liver biopsy, you should:*
a. position him on his right side for 2 hours and promote bed rest for 24 hours.
b. restrict proteins and fluids for 24 hours.
c. assess him for thrombophlebitis and pruritus.
d. tell him he can't have analgesics until after the doctor interprets the test results.

30. *Tell the patient undergoing a cervical punch biopsy that she:*
a. will be hospitalized overnight.
b. should expect heavy bleeding after the procedure and should use tampons as needed.
c. may feel mild discomfort during and after the procedure.
d. should report any foul-smelling vaginal discharge occurring within a week of the procedure.

31. *Which of the following is a disadvantage of ultrasonography?*
a. It doesn't allow an examination of bones or air-filled organs.
b. It can't differentiate between cystic and solid masses.
c. It doesn't allow an evaluation of blood flow in the major blood vessels of the neck and limbs.
d. It can't show motion.

32. *Before your patient undergoes echocardiography, explain to him that:*
a. he may feel some pain but he'll receive an analgesic to relieve it.
b. electrodes will be placed on his chest, wrists, and ankles.
c. the test is safe and painless.
d. the room will be brightly lit and cool.

33. *What should you do if you notice bleeding at the insertion site after cardiac catheterization?*
a. Elevate the patient's limb and notify the doctor.
b. Remove the pressure dressing and ap-

ply firm pressure on the site until the bleeding stops.
c. Obtain vital signs and call for help.
d. Increase the I.V. infusion rate and prepare the patient to return to the cardiac catheterization room.

34. *After bronchoscopy, you should:*
a. keep the patient supine for at least 6 hours.
b. restrict foods, fluids, and oral medications for about 2 hours, until the gag reflex returns.
c. encourage immediate fluid intake.

d. encourage the patient to cough forcefully and frequently.

35. *Before your patient undergoes a liver-spleen scan, you should explain that he:*
a. may feel some discomfort as the transducer passes over his abdomen.
b. will receive an I.V. injection of a radioactive agent 10 to 15 minutes before the scan.
c. will have to stay in bed for 24 hours after the scan.
d. should avoid caffeinated beverages for 10 hours after the test.

ANSWERS

1. b	**6.** c	**11.** d	**16.** b	**21.** b	**26.** a	**31.** a
2. a	**7.** a	**12.** c	**17.** a	**22.** c	**27.** c	**32.** c
3. c	**8.** b	**13.** a	**18.** d	**23.** b	**28.** d	**33.** b
4. b	**9.** d	**14.** c	**19.** b	**24.** a	**29.** a	**34.** b
5. d	**10.** a	**15.** d	**20.** a	**25.** c	**30.** c	**35.** b

APPENDIX
AND
INDEX

Drug interference with test results

Drugs can interfere with the results of laboratory tests in two ways. A drug in a blood or urine specimen may interact with the chemicals used in the laboratory test, causing a false result. Or a drug may cause a physiologic change in the patient, resulting in an actual increased or decreased blood or urine level of the substance being tested. This chart identifies drugs that can cause these two types of interference in some common blood and urine tests.

TEST	CHEMICAL REACTION	PHYSIOLOGIC CHANGE	
		Increased test values	Decreased test values
alkaline phosphatase	• albumin • fluorides	• anticonvulsants • hepatotoxic drugs	• clofibrate
ammonia, blood		• acetazolamide • alcohol • ammonium chloride • asparaginase • barbiturates • diuretics, loop and thiazide	• kanamycin, oral • lactulose • neomycin, oral • potassium salts
amylase, serum	• chloride salts • fluorides	• asparaginase • cholinergic agents • contraceptives, oral • contrast media with iodine • drugs inducing acute pancreatitis: azathioprine, corticosteroids, loop and thiazide diuretics • methyldopa • narcotics	
aspartate aminotransferase	• erythromycin • methyldopa	• cholinergic agents • hepatotoxic drugs • opium alkaloids	
bilirubin, serum	• ascorbic acid • dextran • epinephrine • pindolol	• hemolytic agents • hepatotoxic drugs • methyldopa • rifampin	• barbiturates
blood urea nitrogen	• chloral hydrate • chloramphenicol • streptomycin	• anabolic steroids • nephrotoxic drugs	• tetracyclines
calcium, serum	• aspirin • heparin • hydralazine • sulfisoxazole	• asparaginase • calcium salts • diuretics, loop and thiazide • lithium • thyroid hormones • vitamin D	• acetazolamide • anticonvulsants • calcitonin • cisplatin • contraceptives, oral • corticosteroids • laxatives • magnesium salts • plicamycin

Drug interference with test results *(continued)*

TEST	CHEMICAL REACTION	PHYSIOLOGIC CHANGE	
		Increased test values	Decreased test values
chloride, serum		• acetazolamide • androgens • estrogens • nonsteroidal anti-inflammatory drugs	• corticosteroids • diuretics, loop and thiazide
cholesterol, serum	• androgens • aspirin • corticosteroids • nitrates • phenothiazines • vitamin D	• beta-adrenergic blocking agents • contraceptives, oral • corticosteroids • diuretics, thiazide • phenothiazines • sulfonamides	• androgens • captopril • chlorpropamide • cholestyramine • clofibrate • colestipol • haloperidol • neomycin, oral
creatine phosphokinase (CPK)		• aminocaproic acid • amphotericin B • chlorthalidone • clofibrate • ethanol, chronic use	
creatinine, serum	• cefoxitin (Jaffe method) • cephalothin • flucytosine	• cimetidine • nephrotoxic drugs	
glucose, serum	• acetaminophen • ascorbic acid (urine) • cephalosporins (urine)	• antidepressants, tricyclic • beta-adrenergic blocking agents • corticosteroids • dextrothyroxine • diazoxide • diuretics, loop and thiazide • epinephrine • estrogens • isoniazid • lithium • phenothiazines • phenytoin • salicylates, toxic levels • thiabendazole	• acetaminophen • alcohol • anabolic steroids • clofibrate • disopyramide • gemfibrozil • monoamine oxidase (MAO) inhibitors • pentamidine
magnesium, serum		• lithium • magnesium salts	• alcohol • aminoglycosides • amphotericin B • calcium salts • cisplatin • digitalis glycosides, toxic levels • diuretics, loop and thiazide

(continued)

Drug interference with test results *(continued)*

TEST	CHEMICAL REACTION	PHYSIOLOGIC CHANGE	
		Increased test values	**Decreased test values**
phosphates, serum		• vitamin D, excessive amounts	• antacids, phosphate-binding (such as aluminum phosphate gel) • mannitol
potassium, serum		• aminocaproic acid • angiotensin-converting enzyme (ACE) inhibitors • antineoplastic agents • diuretics, potassium-sparing • isoniazid • lithium • mannitol • nephrotoxic drugs • succinylcholine	• ammonium chloride • amphotericin B • corticosteroids • diuretics, potassium-wasting • glucose • insulin • laxatives • penicillins, extended-spectrum • salicylates
protein, serum		• anabolic steroids • corticosteroids • phenazopyridine	• contraceptives, oral • estrogens • hepatotoxic drugs
protein, urine	• aminoglycosides • cephalosporins • contrast media with iodine • magnesium sulfate, large doses • miconazole • nafcillin • phenazopyridine • sulfonamides • tolbutamide • tolmetin	• cephalosporins • contrast media with iodine • corticosteroids • nafcillin • nephrotoxic drugs • sulfonamides	
prothrombin time		• anticoagulants • asparaginase • aspirin • azathioprine • cefamandole • cefoperazone • cephalothin • chloramphenicol • cholestyramine • colestipol • cyclophosphamide • hepatotoxic drugs • moxalactam • propylthiouracil • quinidine • quinine • sulfonamides • tetracyclines	• anabolic steroids • contraceptives, oral • estrogens • vitamin K

Drug interference with test results *(continued)*

TEST	CHEMICAL REACTION	PHYSIOLOGIC CHANGE	
		Increased test values	Decreased test values
sodium, serum		• anabolic steroids • clonidine • contraceptives, oral • corticosteroids • diazoxide • estrogens • guanabenz • guanadrel • guanethidine • methyldopa • nonsteroidal anti-inflammatory drugs • sulfonylureas	• ammonium chloride • carbamazepine • desmopressin • diuretics • lypressin • vasopressin
uric acid, serum	• ascorbic acid • caffeine • levodopa • theophylline	• acetazolamide • alcohol • cisplatin • diazoxide • diuretics • epinephrine • ethambutol • levodopa • niacin	• acetohexamide • allopurinol • clofibrate • contrast media with iodine • diflunisal • glucose infusions • guaifenesin • phenothiazines • phenylbutazone • salicylates, small doses • uricosuric agents

INDEX

i refers to an illustration; t refers to a table